PERSPECTIVES ON WRITING
Series Editor, Susan H. McLeod

PERSPECTIVES ON WRITING
Series Editor, Susan H. McLeod

The Perspectives on Writing series addresses writing studies in a broad sense. Consistent with the wide ranging approaches characteristic of teaching and scholarship in writing across the curriculum, the series presents works that take divergent perspectives on working as a writer, teaching writing, administering writing programs, and studying writing in its various forms.

The WAC Clearinghouse and Parlor Press are collaborating so that these books will be widely available through free digital distribution and low-cost print editions. The publishers and the Series editor are teachers and researchers of writing, committed to the principle that knowledge should freely circulate. We see the opportunities that new technologies have for further democratizing knowledge. And we see that to share the power of writing is to share the means for all to articulate their needs, interest, and learning into the great experiment of literacy.

Recent Books in the Series

Sarah Allen, *Beyond Argument: Essaying as a Practice of (Ex)Change* (2015)
Steven J. Corbett, *Beyond Dichotomy: Synergizing Writing Center and Classroom Pedagogies* (2015)
Tara Roeder and Roseanne Gatto (Eds.), *Critical Expressivism: Theory and Practice in the Composition Classroom* (2015)
Terry Myers Zawacki and Michelle Cox, *WAC and Second-Language Writers: Research Towards Linguistically and Culturally Inclusive Programs and Practices* (2014)
Charles Bazerman, *A Rhetoric of Literate Action: Literate Action Volume 1* (2013)
Charles Bazerman, *A Theory of Literate Action: Literate Action Volume 2* (2013)
Katherine V. Wills and Rich Rice (Eds.), *ePortfolio Performance Support Systems: Constructing, Presenting, and Assessing Portfolios* (2013)
Mike Duncan and Star Medzerian Vanguri (Eds.), *The Centrality of Style* (2013)
Chris Thaiss, Gerd Bräuer, Paula Carlino, Lisa Ganobcsik-Williams, and Aparna Sinha (Eds.), *Writing Programs Worldwide: Profiles of Academic Writing in Many Places* (2012)
Andy Kirkpatrick and Zhichang Xu, *Chinese Rhetoric and Writing: An Introduction for Language Teachers* (2012)

YOGA MINDS, WRITING BODIES: CONTEMPLATIVE WRITING PEDAGOGY

Christy I. Wenger

The WAC Clearinghouse
wac.colostate.edu
Fort Collins, Colorado

Parlor Press
www.parlorpress.com
Anderson, South Carolina

The WAC Clearinghouse, Fort Collins, Colorado 80523-1052
Parlor Press, 3015 Brackenberry Drive, Anderson, South Carolina 29621

© 2015 by Christy I. Wenger. This work is licensed under a Creative Commons Attribution-NonCommercial-NoDerivatives 4.0 International.

Printed in the United States of America

Library of Congress Cataloging-in-Publication Data

Wenger, Christy I., 1982-
　Yoga minds, writing bodies : contemplative writing pedagogy / Christy I. Wenger.
　　　pages cm. -- (Perspectives on writing)
　Includes bibliographical references.
　ISBN 978-1-60235-660-3 (pbk. : acid-free paper) -- ISBN 978-1-60235-661-0 (hardcover : acid-free paper)
　1. English language--Composition and exercises--Study and teaching. 2. Mind and body. 3. Self in literature. 4. Yoga. I. Title.
　PE1404.W4546 2015
　808'.04207--dc23
　　　　　　　　　　　　2015006893

Copyeditor: Don Donahue
Designer: Tara Reeser
Series Editor: Susan H. McLeod

This book is printed on acid-free paper.

The WAC Clearinghouse supports teachers of writing across the disciplines. Hosted by Colorado State University, it brings together scholarly journals and book series as well as resources for teachers who use writing in their courses. This book is available in digital format for free download at http://wac.colostate.edu.

Parlor Press, LLC is an independent publisher of scholarly and trade titles in print and multimedia formats. This book is available in print and digital formats from Parlor Press at http://www.parlorpress.com. For submission information or to find out about Parlor Press publications, write to Parlor Press, 3015 Brackenberry Drive, Anderson, South Carolina 29621, or email editor@parlorpress.com.

PREFACE

> In the beginning, there is no substitute for sweat.
> —BKS Iyengar, *Light on Life*

I take a hard look in the mirror, noting my yoga pants and sneakers. As someone who prefers to dress business casual for teaching, this outfit is a deviation that feels both exciting, because it's freeingly comfortable, and a bit scary. I chose my loose-fitted yoga pants carefully today, avoiding the skin-tight pair I regularly wear to the yoga studio. Through my slow development as a yogi, I've learned that to understand your body, you have to see it; to see it clearly, you have to claim it. It's hard to see if your knee is lined up over your big toe, for example, if that knee is swallowed up by fabric. Tighter fits allow for better alignment assessment and easier movement in yoga. While my tight pants have a practical purpose, then, that they've come to rest in my closet is just one indication of how far I'd come in letting go of my body self-consciousness and claiming my body as it is. As a yogi, I understand these actions of giving myself over to my practice—worrying less about others' perceptions of my body and more about my own sense of embodiment—as a sign of growth. As a writing teacher-cum-yogi about to bring these two worlds together, however, I proceed with measure. Still standing in front of my mirror, I move my arms up and down to make sure my top stays in place. I plan to complete today's yoga practice with my first-year writing students and don't relish the idea of them seeing unveiled any part of my body that would be normally clothed.

Abandoning body self-consciousness is, I have found, is a very slow process. Much like gaining confidence as a writer.

Before I can turn away from my reflection, I see the wide eyes of someone not only excited but also a little afraid. I must admit to myself that I'm wondering if my first-year writing students will revolt after today's yoga practice with my Iyengar teacher and me. I am worried about what will happen when I display what I could never hide but for years tried to ignore in the classroom: my own young, female body. As a neophyte scholar, I only have about a decade on most of my students, and I worry that acknowledgement of my flesh could disrupt my "teacherly" authority, sending the class on a collision course toward chaos. Of course as a yogi, I realize this is unlikely and desire to push through the learned fear until it is a distant memory. My experience as a "writing yogi" is why I am doing this, giving my students the chance to incorporate yoga into their writing processes as I've done with great success. I've reached this moment because I can no longer think of writing and yoga as separate processes, linked as they are by a common core of mindfulness. But, I still can't keep the old, learned panic from nipping at me.

My students filtered into the dance studio of the campus dance studio slowly. Most took my injunction to wear loose-fitting, comfortable "workout" clothes seriously. Though, two male students came in jeans and t-shirts, perhaps to suggest their lack of enthusiasm. Everyone looked around nervously, spotting the huge stack of folded blankets on the side of the room, blankets my yoga teacher, Holly, and I and her two assistants lugged up in huge, black trash bags to the third floor of my campus' gym. In the nervous energy that accumulated before my students showed up for class, I neatly folded those trash bags and placed them in a pile behind the blankets; the challenge of folding plastic was a welcome distraction to what would come next. As for the blankets themselves, Holly was adamant that we provide props for my students so as to better accommodate the restorative poses with which we'd start and end class. Indeed, if she'd had her way, we would have moved the bricks and straps from her studio across town to this room as well. The copious use of props is a feature of the kind of yoga we'd do today. Iyengar yoga can accommodate a range of students' needs and flexibilities by modifying poses using props. Among other reasons, it is such adaptability that makes this Hatha approach a friendly one for the writing classroom.

Today was the day all our joint planning would hopefully pay off, and Holly and I were committed to giving my students a taste of "real" yoga even as we strived for a structure that wouldn't be intimidating and that would fit organically into the overall goals of my writing class. My writing students were prepared for today's "yoga for writers" practice from the day they stepped foot in my course. They knew that their body blogs and our exploration of the physical demands of the writing process would eventually bring us to this first day of practicing yoga together as a class. After exploring the importance of our writing bodies for the first quarter of the semester, we would finally be learning yoga so we could experiment with integrating *asanas*, or poses, in our composing processes from this point on. Today, we would be led by a certified instructor, my own yoga teacher, who generously offered to teach my writing class a series of yoga poses that we chose together, carefully sequenced and then dubbed a "yoga for writers" practice.

By my eyes and their own accounts (which I would read later in their blogs), my students seemed wary as they entered the room. They immediately took in the presence of Holly and her assistants—one male and one female. I hoped the male assistant served as an important reminder for my male students, especially the jean-clad ones, that yoga wasn't "girly" or inherently emasculating. Since young men at my university tended to approach yoga as a form of women's exercise, I'd previously mentioned that the yoga classes I take right outside of the university's bounds are populated with just as many male as female yogis and talked about how professional football players were using yoga as a way to develop body awareness, strength and flexibility. My students and I had eventually come together over the irony that a practice dominated by men in India is so differently characterized by American youth culture. Noting the assistants, students looked back to me for reassurance. Their eyes seemed to say, "I guess we really are doing yoga in our class today." I smiled hopefully at them.

My students look apprehensive, but I believe myself to be the most nervous person in the room. I worry that despite my attempts to prepare them and funnel our class toward this very moment, they will not discover even a degree of embodied awareness today. If they can't make the connections between yoga and writing on their own and through their individual bodies, I can only pray they won't write me off along with our practice. What if they start to view me as some "crunchy," new-age hippie wasting their time? How can I finish the semester without incident if my students no longer respect me or my authority as their composition instructor? I realize in a moment of clarity that an anxious teacher isn't the most convincing, so I try to swallow my nerves and to smile confidently at them as they enter the room. One by one, they look to me for reassurance, and I find myself nodding and telling them to take off their shoes and grab a blanket, trying to draw strength from routine. This is, after all, how Holly has run all of her yoga classes, so it has been my routine as a student of hers. My roles as student and teacher merge as my worlds collide.

I hoped that our mindful preparation and organization as well as Holly's evident and serious passion for yoga would help students leave behind prior judgment and would mediate their trepidations with a sense of adventure. I had great faith in Holly's no-nonsense approach. It was tempered by genuine friendliness and a desire to share her practice with others that was infectious to me as a yoga student. I hoped that her fire-and-ice combination would keep my students on task and prevent them from goofing off. Holly began by asking students how they were feeling, noting that many looked exhausted. I wouldn't normally ask students how tired they were feeling, so this question surprised me for a moment. And, even if my students acknowledged their exhaustion in those chatty moments before the day's lesson had begun, I wouldn't necessarily think to give them a moment to reconnect and revive themselves for the tasks that lie ahead during our class time together. But, this is how Holly started. As my students explained their hectic weeks of athletic practices, late nights studying for tests in the library and writing papers, I began to notice just how much weariness they wore on their faces and the exhaustion with which they seemed to carry their bodies. I couldn't help but wonder how many times in previous classes I'd misread exhaustion for disengagement.

Holly promised students that our practice would help with their exhaustion. Already being listened to, they responded in turn and took Holly's instruction to fold up their blankets in thirds as she was. They copied her model of the first pose, *savasana,* which she showed them by lying on the floor in a supine position with arms and legs relaxed to the sides of the body.[1] To encourage students' energetic involvement and their full presence during our practice of the more active poses or *asanas,* we started students in this restorative pose, which is meant to calm the mind and quiet the body. If their responses to Holly's first question were an appropriate gauge, my students were in great need of momentary physical rest and a stilling of their minds.

Students relaxed into *savasana* with a blanket folded in thirds beneath and between their shoulder blades to help open up their chests. In yoga, chest openers are not only meant to be physically restorative, as a way to counter the rounded shoulders cultivated by too many hours in front of the computer or sitting in chairs with poor posture but are also thought to open up the heart and mind to new ideas. Because yoga sees the metaphoric and physical as interconnected, it is understood that as we open up physically, we are less likely to make snap judgments and are more likely to approach ourselves and others with balance, compassion and non-violence, called *ahimsa*. Of course, on a literal level balance and openness are important for my students, many of whom never practiced yoga before and would have to be patient with their tight bodies; they would have to let go of debilitating judgments if they found their peers to be more limber than themselves, for instance. Further, on an imaginative level, I hoped students would be influenced by this opening pose to give our practice a fair chance and not immediately judge it as a poor use for a class meeting. Happily, students' sighs as they settled into this pose were a testament to the relief they felt at being given a chance to relax before asked to exert themselves once more for a teacher's demands.

Moving them into an easy seated, cross-legged pose from *savasana,* we asked students to set an intention or *sankulpa* for their practice, noting that this intention was to guide and give meaning to their movements. We explained that this was like having a goal when writing a paper. Intentions remind students to listen to their bodies as they move them in new and different ways, promoting focus and giving them a feeling of purpose to carry into their practice of yoga—or writing. Setting an intention is a conscious way to bridge the mind and body's intelligence and can help students learn to connect feelings and thoughts, increasing awareness of both. Drawing inward for a moment consequently helps develop self-reflection and increases flexibility. This practice of reconnecting with ourselves is understood to give measure to our actions, teaching us that we can control our response to stimuli by listening to our bodies and using our energy productively and not for unthinkingly reacting to everything that comes our way. The practice of choosing what we react to is a ritual we would later use to support curiosity and engagement when tackling how to integrate outside sources and differing perspectives in our writing.

Before I can think much about what my intention should be today, one rises to the surface: I must let go and simply enjoy this experience. I want my being and doing to merge in this intention so that I can find strength and clarity, which I will need in order to know how to bring this practice "home" to our regular classroom meetings after today. As I set this intention, I imagine it arising from my heart and permeating my whole body. When I practice yoga, I like to think of my intentions as beams of light that start in my center and reach to the tips of my toes and fingers so that every cell of my being can find a unity of purpose in the movements to come. Today is no different. As I imagine these beams of light warming me and spreading from my inner body to my outer body, I remember that it is this cultivation of strength from awareness and patience that drew me to yoga in the first place.

To move focus toward self-awareness, we coached students through a process of *pratyahara*, or a slow releasing of tension from the body and consequent withdrawal of the sense organs. We chose to include these practices in order to help students develop a relationship with their bodies that would continue throughout our practice, and later, into their writing. The goal of *pratyahara* is not to ignore everything or to tune it out but to develop calm awareness and concentration in the midst of a distracting world. And because yoga views the body as a mediation point between inner and outer, yoked as we are to other bodies and a material world, drawing inward simultaneously reminds us of the other bodies to which we are connected and creates a felt community between practitioners.

Students then worked on steadying their breath, engaging in *pranayama*, or breath awareness. To keep things simple, Holly asked them to match their outbreaths and in-breaths so as to even them out, bringing peace and promoting focus for the practice to follow. A basic tenant of yoga is that the breath impacts the mind so while Iyengar yoga approaches *pranayama* as a skill of its own right, a separate limb of the eight-fold path of yoga, basic applications of attentive breathing are incorporated from the beginning of *asana* practice. Awareness of the breath is the hinge on which *asanas* turn. When our breathing is even, our thoughts and our actions can be balanced and directed.

With my eyes closed, I breathe slowly, feeling my in-breaths calm me. I hear my out-breaths mingle with my students' who are sitting all around me. At this moment,

I remember why I told Holly I wanted to practice with my class instead of directing up front with her or watching from the sidelines. Not only do I want to help model poses for my students, I also want to testify through my own bodily actions that I am part of our felt community and not an outsider, directing and watching without participating. I hope that our movements together will establish a solidarity and commonality of purpose that will flourish during the remainder of the semester. I hope that we will grow into a contemplative writing community together. For now, I feel I am experiencing a genuine moment of connection; at this moment, I am with my students in ways traditional class structures often make impossible. Here, we are feeling bodies together, breathing and moving our way toward awareness.

CONTENTS

Preface v

Acknowledgments xiii

Introduction: From the Sticky Mat to the Classroom:
Toward Contemplative Writing Pedagogy 3

Chapter One: The Writing Yogi: Lessons for Embodied Change 33

Interchapter One: Using "Body Blogs" to Embody
the Writer's Imagination 59

Chapter Two: Personal Presence, Embodied Empiricism and Resonance
in Contemplative Writing 79

Interchapter Two: Habits of Yoga Minds and Writing Bodies 101

Chapter Three: Situating Feelings in Contemplative Writing Pedagogy 127

Interchapter Three: The Writer's Breath 151

Conclusion: Namaste 177

Notes 179

References 185

Appendix A 193

Appendix B 197

About the Author 199

ACKNOWLEDGMENTS

Raising a child takes a village and so does writing a book. I am thankful for all who comprised my "village;" without them, this book would not have been written.

My deepest gratitude goes to my husband and my mother, both of whom provided me endless cheerleading—and ice cream breaks when needed. Thanks, mom, for raising me to be like you: a strong, confident woman who isn't afraid to take risks. Thanks, Steve, for never doubting what I could accomplish and supporting me all the way through. And, thanks, Nancy, for taking care of Paige so mommy could write.

I thank my departmental colleagues at Shepherd University, many of whom read parts of this text and provided useful feedback for revision during faculty writing group meetings. I also thank the English department faculty and graduate students at my previous institution, Lehigh University, for helping me to build the theoretical foundation and pedagogical practice that serves as the backbone of this book. Of course, I thank my students at both schools for being active participants in my courses and for their willingness to be a part of my project. My students have given me the biggest gift of all: a bounty of greatly reflective writing and honest accounts of their experiences with contemplative pedagogy.

I owe a great deal of gratitude to both my mentors at Lehigh, Barry M. Kroll and Edward Lotto. Both read countless drafts of the earliest stages of this project and pushed me to refine my ideas. They encouraged my pedagogical experimentation and helped me navigate the professional, personal and logistical challenges of getting students to *move* in the classroom. I remain thankful, Barry, for the continued gifts of your time and knowledge.

A special thanks to Laurence Musgrove for helping me with the yoga illustrations throughout the book; you brought my stick figures to life! Thanks also to my peer reviewers and editors. The former offered thoughtful suggestions for revision, which substantially strengthened the final draft of this book, and the latter made the process a smooth one. Editors Sue McLeod, Mike Palmquist and David Blakesley, thanks for making the journey to publication enjoyable.

Not only did my yoga teachers inspire me to write this book, they also helped me implement the contemplative pedagogy I discuss within its pages. Holly, I am deeply grateful that you found my work to join yoga and writing compelling and offered your time and energies to my students. Our many talks on your porch about the philosophy of yoga shaped what this project turned into and gave me the confidence to move forward. Special thanks to Christa and Gena, who have helped me to integrate yoga in my classes at Shepherd. You all have all shaped me as a yogi, which has, in turn, shaped me as a teacher. *Namaste*.

And, to my girls, Jamie, Nikki and Sarah, I offer thanks for years of love and friendship. Thanks for reading drafts, thanks for the free talk therapy and thanks for making me step away from my computer every now and then. In the words of Anne of Green Gables, you are my kindred spirits.

I dedicate this book to my daughter, Paige, who teaches me daily what it means to be mindful and to find joy in the present moment. Mommy loves you.

YOGA MINDS, WRITING BODIES: CONTEMPLATIVE WRITING PEDAGOGY

INTRODUCTION: FROM THE STICKY MAT TO THE CLASSROOM: TOWARD CONTEMPLATIVE WRITING PEDAGOGY

> What we cannot imagine cannot come into being
> —bell hooks, *All About Love*

> The intelligence of the body is a fact. It is real. The intelligence of the brain is only imagination. So the imagination has to be made real. The brain may dream of doing a difficult backbend today, but it cannot force the impossible even on to a willing body. We are always trying to progress, but inner cooperation is essential.
> —BKS Iyengar, *Light on Life*

I move from kneeling on all fours into *Adho Mukha Svanasana*, or downward-facing dog, lifting and straightening my knees and elbows. I exhale along with the rest of my class and try to send this energy down into my hands, pushing each palm evenly onto my mat and pressing the tops of my thighs back in order to descend my heels as close to the floor as possible. Even as I move quietly, my thoughts create a loud frenzy inside my head, destroying the peace for which my *sadhana*, or my practice, aims. This pose frustrates me. I know I'm weak in it, so I begin to question my alignment. As I push my hips back and up, I wonder if my spine is scooping instead of creating a long line. My mind orders my spine to go long, and I think about shifting more weight into my heels. As a result, I forget about my hands and they begin to slide forward, inching their way up to the top of my sticky mat. I wonder with bitterness how terrible my pose looks. This is a genuine concern: with my head down and my eyes staring at my toes, I can't see myself. I begin to wish I could view myself as my teacher and classmates can in order to confirm my fears that I'm doing this pose all wrong. I suppress a sigh and, with no better alternative, begin a silent prayer for the pose to be called to an end.

Instead, I feel hands grab my hips and pull them back. With this action, I feel my heels settle firmly onto my mat. At the same time that she moves me, my yoga instructor, Holly, enjoins me to lift my sitting bones and direct them toward the back of the room.

"Oh. Sorry. I ...." Thoughts racing forward, I fumble to explain my ineptitude.

Holly cuts me off to reply, "No. You need to stop thinking and feel."

Because Holly knows me well, she understands I need to be reminded of this. I know hers isn't a command *never* to think when doing an *asana*, or pose, like *Adho Mukha Svanasana*. Instead, it's a reminder to let my brain and body work *together* in the pose.

This kind of integration is frankly something to which I am not accustomed as an academic and a compositionist. Jane Tompkins may have written Me and My Shadow decades ago, singling out the professional discourse community of composition studies and indicting its propensity to separate our personal, material realities from our professional voices, but hers is a reality I share years later. Nevertheless as a yogi and increasingly as a feminist and a writing teacher, claiming my body is a move I know I need to make for growth. The above example from my yoga practice makes this lesson clear. Rather than trying to force my body into confused compliance as I was in my frustration with downward-facing dog, Holly's message was that I needed to listen to it. When I could *feel* my hips shift back and down, when I could find a balance between the agency of my body and the directives of my mind, I would have little need for my earlier out-of-body desire to see myself; instead, I could use these embodied, critical feelings to work toward a better pose and, therein, a more holistic sense of self, a contemplative awareness of my subjectivity. But to achieve this end, I first must relax my habit of trying to control my body with my mind and, through awareness, learn to work with my physical body's organic intelligence and to respect it as a site of knowledge. When I can do this, I will improve my mindfulness of how knowledge is created and embodied in both processes around which I structure so much of my life: yoga and writing.

SETTING INTENTIONS AND PRACTICING THEORY

I begin this introduction with a recent experience from my Iyengar yoga class in order to frame my *sankalpa*, the Sanskrit word for intention, in this project: namely, exploring the consequences of stepping away from pedagogies that overlook students' and teachers' embodiments and toward contemplative writing pedagogies that view the body as a lived site of knowledge and not, primarily, as a discursive text. In response to higher education's growing interest in contemplative education and a reaffirmed commitment within composition studies to create pedagogies that facilitate a meaningful transfer of skills, this book argues that contemplative practices should be integrated in our college writing curricula. Using the embodied insights from contemplative practices like yoga, meditation and the martial arts, among others, and fusing them with a traditional curriculum is what distinguishes contemplative education from other learning methods. Professor at Amherst University and Director of the Mind and Life Institute, Arthur Zajonc, notes that contemplative pedagogies offer teachers "a wide range of educational methods that support the development of student attention, emotional balance, empathetic connection, compassion, and altruistic behavior, while also providing new pedagogical techniques that support creativity and the learning of course content" (2010, p. 83). Writing pedagogies that integrate contemplative practices are concrete examples of how we might forward—with difference—recent attention to embodied rhetorics. For, contemplative pedagogies not only self-consciously take up the body, but they also direct focus to *mindfulness*, an embodied intervention that creates a rich source of practice and theory which can be used to transform the work completed in our college writing classrooms and the ways that work is transferred to other writing environments.

The rhetorical primacy of the body is guaranteed within contemplative pedagogy by mindfulness, or moment-to-moment awareness. Mindfulness is the practice of slowing down and paying close attention to the present moment. We practice mindfulness when each "thought feeling or sensation that arises in the attentional field is acknowledged and accepted as it is" (Bishop et al., n.d., p. 8). Rather than over-identifying with or immediately reacting to thoughts and feelings as they arise, the practitioner of mindfulness creates a critical distance, a space between perception and response, that allows for eventual, intentional response as opposed to automatic, unthinking and habitual reaction (Bishop et al., n.d., p. 9). As my reader will see in the coming chapters, mindfulness forces us to be responsive to the sensations of our bodies and our corresponding feelings; it roots us in the present moment so that we may more consciously shape our future actions. Because it encourages careful consideration and choice, mindfulness fosters in writers the kind of rhetorical responsibility characteristic of embodied approaches to writing and rhetoric.

While embodied rhetorics remain a relatively new area of interest for the field of composition studies, some beginning explorations have started to document the changes that occur when awareness of the organic body productively interrupts our professional writing (Jane Hindman's Making Writing Matter), reflections on our teaching (William Banks' Written Through the Body; Tina

Kazan's Dancing Bodies) and our understanding of literacy as primarily verbal (Kristie Fleckenstein's *Embodied Literacies*). While no two embodied writing pedagogies are exactly alike, they are all united by the common purpose of inserting the body into education by self-consciously attending to the somatics of learning and teaching. Debra Hawhee points out that recent interest in embodied pedagogy actually returns us to an ancient connection between rhetorical and athletic training. Hawhee reveals that

> sophistic pedagogy displayed a curious syncretism between athletics and rhetoric, a particular crossover in pedagogical practices and learning styles, a crossover that contributed to the development of rhetoric as a *bodily art:* an art learned, practiced, and performed by and with the body as well as the mind. (2002, p. 144)

Whether we view them as contemporary movements or renewals of classic paradigms, these pedagogies have effectively shifted our focus to the material bodies of the students and professionals involved in the act of writing and away from a strict theoretical discourse of the subject who is written.

Raul Sanchez overviews the history of this shift in his recent *College English* article, Outside the Text: Retheorizing Empiricism and Identity. Sanchez argues that the defining feature of the postmodern moment, which he situates in the 1980s to 1990s within composition studies, was an emphasis on "the subject," a theoretical term that questioned the validity of "the writer," a term rooted in realist materiality: "[t]he writer and the subject, then, have not been interchangeable: the latter remains a figure with which to theorize systematically, while the former is encountered materially and individually" (2012, p. 235). Noting we are now past postmodernism, Sanchez claims we are once again asking ourselves what's "outside" of writing. Sanchez' central query establishes recent investigations of embodied writing—and this project's focus on contemplative writing, arguably a richer alternative—as part of a contemporary, historical movement to validate "commonsense materiality" (2012, p. 235).

Indeed, embodied writing's exigency typically springs from the postmodernist zeal to "read away" or narratize the organic body by understanding discursive consciousness as *the* site of struggle and agency (see, for instance, Fleckenstein's Writing Bodies). To look for a paradigmatic example of what happens when a pedagogy validates subjects and not writers, we need to look no further than James Berlin's social epistemicism. Critical pedagogies like social epistemicism have justified the erasure of the organic body by insisting that our coming to consciousness *is* our coming to language, a powerful move that validates the kind of rhetorical analysis so key to our field. With its attention on the writer, Sanchez' essay marks the new spaces opening up in our field for teaching methods that neither ignore the shaping powers of language nor condemn the body to a linguistic prison, classified as a trope. It is within this space that I insert contemplative writing pedagogy.

By starting from the perspective of the body, contemplative writing pedagogy represents a hopeful alternative that shares a fundamental goal with approaches under the larger umbrella of embodied rhetorics: to cultivate an understanding of embodiment as more than simply a conceptual framework (even if it may be, in part, this too) but also as a lived, fleshy reality. It is this fleshy reality my students and I encountered in our first practice of yoga together, which I narrate in my preface. Tompkins, perhaps one of the first in composition studies to gain notoriety for her enactment of embodied writing before it was even labeled as such, argues that the separation of the personal from the professional is due to interdisciplinary trends within the professoriate that insist on objectivity as a prerequisite for responsibility and truth. Being schooled within a system that places value on the "life of the mind" over the supposed banality of her flesh creates tension between the particularities of embodied experience and the promise of transcendence in Tompkins' real life. For instance, Tompkins cannot reconcile her academic persona with her personal embodied reality. She describes in *A Life in School* an inverse relation between her achievements in school and her body's physical sufferings, including wetting her bed and developing physical ailments for no explainable reasons. In Me and My Shadow, Tompkins questions this relationship by inserting her lived body into her narrative, saying, for example, that as she writes, she is "thinking about going to the bathroom. But not going yet" (1987, p. 173). Such a fleshy interjection startles readers and reminds us that when objectivity is construed as an erasure of the body, the split between the personal and academic becomes a metonym for the hierarchical divide between the body and mind. Tompkin's unapologetic reference to her body doesn't "belong" in academic writing because it breaks the rules of "mind over matter"—even if readers identify with the reality of her observations given their own lived experiences. Precisely because they disrupt, hers become examples of the body's refusal to be ignored despite our best attempts at theorizing it away.

It is not surprising that female scholars like Tompkins have been at the forefront of critiques that center on the dangers of a disembodied academe. Historically, women have not been able to elide their embodiment because patriarchal systems have simply reduced them to their bodies, allowing men to be associated with the transcendent mind. Because patriarchal power often rests on the ability to cast women solely as body objects, academic feminism has been wary to claim the reality of the physical body lest it naturalize that body once more. Feminism's struggle with the organic body was the subject of a talk by Toril Moi who visited my former university as I worked on this project in the spring of 2010. Despite Moi's warnings, a struggle it remains: feminism has placed women's bodies at the center of political and theoretical discussion and scholarship since its beginnings, but it too often continues to do so without the aim of claiming the organic body's ordinary materiality, its integrity beyond language.

No feminist writing pedagogy can stand outside the influence of Judith Butler's work to rhetoricize gender.[2] But just as Butler's work has helped shape what it means to theorize and to practice feminism in our composition classrooms, resulting in popular field readers like *Feminism and Composition: A Critical Sourcebook*, it has also served to naturalize the textualization of the body. Susan Bordo, pithily capturing the problem of using Butler to drive our pedagogies, writes, "Butler's world is one in which language swallows everything up, voraciously, a theoretical pasta-machine through which the categories of competing frameworks are pressed and reprocessed as "tropes" (1993, p. 291). Focused more on what we gain (attention to the social construction of gender and its performance) than what we lose (attention to the physical world and the material body), feminist sociologist Alexandra Howson argues that we have too heavily relied on these tropes. As a result, "the body appears in much feminist theory as an ethereal presence, a fetishized concept that has become detached and totalizing for the interpretive communities it serves" (2005, p. 3). Howson tasks herself the project of corporalizing gender studies and exploring the particularity of embodiment as applied to her field, which shares with our own an interest in real people and authentic spaces of living and learning.

By dialoguing feminism with contemplative pedagogy, I hope to expand the spirit of Howson's project and make it applicable to our field. The abstraction of the body has left personal experiences and pragmatics of embodiment felt by individual student and teacher bodies devalued for the construction and representation of corporeality as a social performance. To claim these embodied experiences as "personal" does not do enough to insist on their material reality—a reality that extends beyond semiotics. Compositionists, especially those interested in feminisms, have lost too much by resting our critique there. To the revaluation of the personal that Tompkins started years ago, I argue that feminist compositionists must add an unabashed focus on organic embodiment via the contemplative. In this book, I will examine how the metonymic confusion of the body and the personal in composition studies, while pragmatic and understandable, has tended to stunt conversations about the body by simply casting it under the net of the personal, thereby entrenching it in the circular, pedagogical debate between personal writing and critical writing, neither of which can support a serious investigation of matter.

Contemplative pedagogy moves us beyond these divisions and gives us a third possibility. In contemplative traditions like yoga, embodiment becomes the means of knowing, feeling and making sense of the world and not just a physical enactment of social forces. Contemplative pedagogies are distinctive in that they capture the importance of felt knowledge as a creative force on both content and process levels without capitulating to solipsistic or essentialist-expressivist notions of singular embodiment. The kind of felt knowledge to which I refer certainly encompasses Sondra Perl's exploration of Eugene Gendlin's felt sense, or the "body's knowledge before it's articulated in words" (2004, p. 1), but expands beyond it too, as it doesn't preclude discursive knowingness nor need it be built entirely on intuition. In contemplative writing pedagogy as in yoga, the body and mind are both agentive and creative forces, companionate in relation to one another. The personal narrative I relate to begin my introduction captures this intelligent interdependence. Respecting the natural or organic body does not mean we ignore the dynamism of nature or the shaping powers of culture: just because I accept my body as real doesn't mean I can't also resist notions of authentic feminine essence on and off my sticky mat.

As far back as the 1980s, James Moffett drew our attention in his Writing, Inner Speech and Meditation to the ways Eastern practices like meditation could sustain the development of somatic awareness where our own cultural practices fell short. More recently, Mary Rose O'Reilley has argued that the contemplative tradition of claiming silence central to Buddhism and present in Quaker rituals can be of value to our classrooms. Marianthe Karanikas claims as well that "meditative exercises can help students uncover their tacit assumptions, become aware of their biases, and begin to act mindfully in any number of situations" (1997, p. 161) based on her experiments in the technical writing classroom. My embodied experiences have also led me to contemplative pedagogies. Zajonc has called such growing interest in the contemplative a "quiet revolution in higher education" (2010, p. 83). I am not alone, then, in my interest to explore what contemplative pedagogies might add to our classrooms. Our current decade has seen an explosion of interest in the contemplative within academic circles. Here are just a few of interest to those of us who teach:

- In 2001, the Mindfulness in Education Network (MiEN) was established with the purpose of "facilitat[ing] communication among all educators, parents, students and any others interested in promoting contemplative practice (mindfulness) in educational settings," according to its website. MiEN sponsors annual conferences on mindfulness

in education and maintains an active listserv of over 1,000 educators interested in sharing mindful approaches to teaching.
- In 2003, the Garrison Institute was founded as a non-profit, non-sectarian organization committed to exploring "the intersection of contemplation and engaged action in the world" and education ("Envisioning," 2009). In 2005, the institute released a report mapping the use of contemplative educational programs and presented this "Mapping Project" at the first Garrison Institute Symposium on Contemplation and Education in April. In 2008, the institute issued a report on the growing trends of contemplative education as discussed at their education leadership forum held the same year.
- In 2006, Teacher's College Record published a special issue on contemplative practices in higher education, which grew out of a national conference at Teacher's College, Columbia University, highlighting the growing inclusion not only of these practices within individual classrooms but also the building of centers and programs for mindfulness on campuses ("Contemplative Practices and Education," 2006).
- In May 2008, The Association for the Contemplative Mind in Higher Education (ACMHE) was launched. Starting as an "Academic Program" of the Association for the Contemplative Mind in Society and after ten years of administering fellowships to contemplative educators, the ACMHE grew into a program of its own standing. Today, the program is a "multidisciplinary, not-for-profit, professional academic association with a membership of educators, scholars, and administrators in higher education," which "promotes the emergence of a broad culture of contemplation in the academy by connecting a network of leading institutions and academics committed to the recovery and development of the contemplative dimension of teaching, learning and knowing," according to its website (Zajonc, n.d).

Important as the above milestones are in establishing the prominence of contemplative education as a central query and legitimate practice for those of us situated within higher education, they are nowhere near the only that might be cited. Large initiatives like the ACMHE and the MiEN network and more local, institutional programs like Brown's thriving Contemplative Studies Initiative are just a few of the many testimonies we have on how popular and invasive the recent move toward contemplative education has become within American universities. These programs and initiatives echo a larger cultural uptake of the contemplative, a critical mass of public discourse and awareness about contemplative practice. Take yoga, for instance. In 2008, 15.8 million

Americans practiced yoga and spent around $5.7 billion on yoga classes and related products, according to a study done by *The Yoga Journal*. This level of spending amounted to an increase of 87% as compared to the journal's previous study, conducted in 2004 (Macy, 2008). Such findings hold up locally, I've found. In my own small department, there are three of us who regularly practice yoga, and my small university downtown area has two yoga studios (though no stoplights).

Aside from following larger cultural trends, academic interest in the contemplative has also been driven by new scientific evidence that testifies to the beneficial psychophysiological effects of practices like mediation and yoga. Growing acceptance and inclusion of the contemplative within the university "is happening, not coincidentally [then], as the scientific research on mindfulness is expanding and producing results relevant to teaching, learning and knowing," notes Mirabai Bush, cofounder of ACMHE (2011, p. 183). And, this expansion is itself notable: "[o]ver the last twenty years, there has been an exponential increase in research ... from some eighty published papers in 1990 to over six hundred in 2000" (Smalley & Winston, 2010, p. 2).

Bush's comments remind us that the focus on mindfulness is the key to contemplative education, not which methods are used to cultivate it. Contemplative teachers willingly model mindfulness for their students and coach students to use mindfulness to enhance their creativity, attentional focus, awareness of others and proprioperception. In this book, I am most interested in contemplative pedagogies that incorporate yoga as the primary means of developing mindfulness of the body as an epistemic origin; though, the insights contained within can be cultivated using a variety of other contemplative practices and can be easily translated to other contemplative pedagogies provided that they follow the tenants of mindfulness. See figure 1: "The Tree of Contemplative Practices" for just some of the many practices that engage us in mindfulness training. Barry M. Kroll, for instance, provides a complementary but different approach in his recent, *The Open Hand: Arguing as An Art of Peace*. Kroll details his creation of a freshman seminar devoted to the instruction of non-adversarial methods of argumentation—deliberative, conciliatory and integrative—through, in large part, the incorporation of contemplative practices and meditative arts. He uses Aikido as a way to teach students how they might "cultivate awareness and equanimity in the midst of conflict" (2013, p. 3). Kroll goes to the movements of Aikido as a humble practitioner and introduces those as "a physical analogy for the tactics of arguing" (2013, p. 12) in much the same way that I introduce yoga to first-year students as a means of reframing and navigating the writing process.

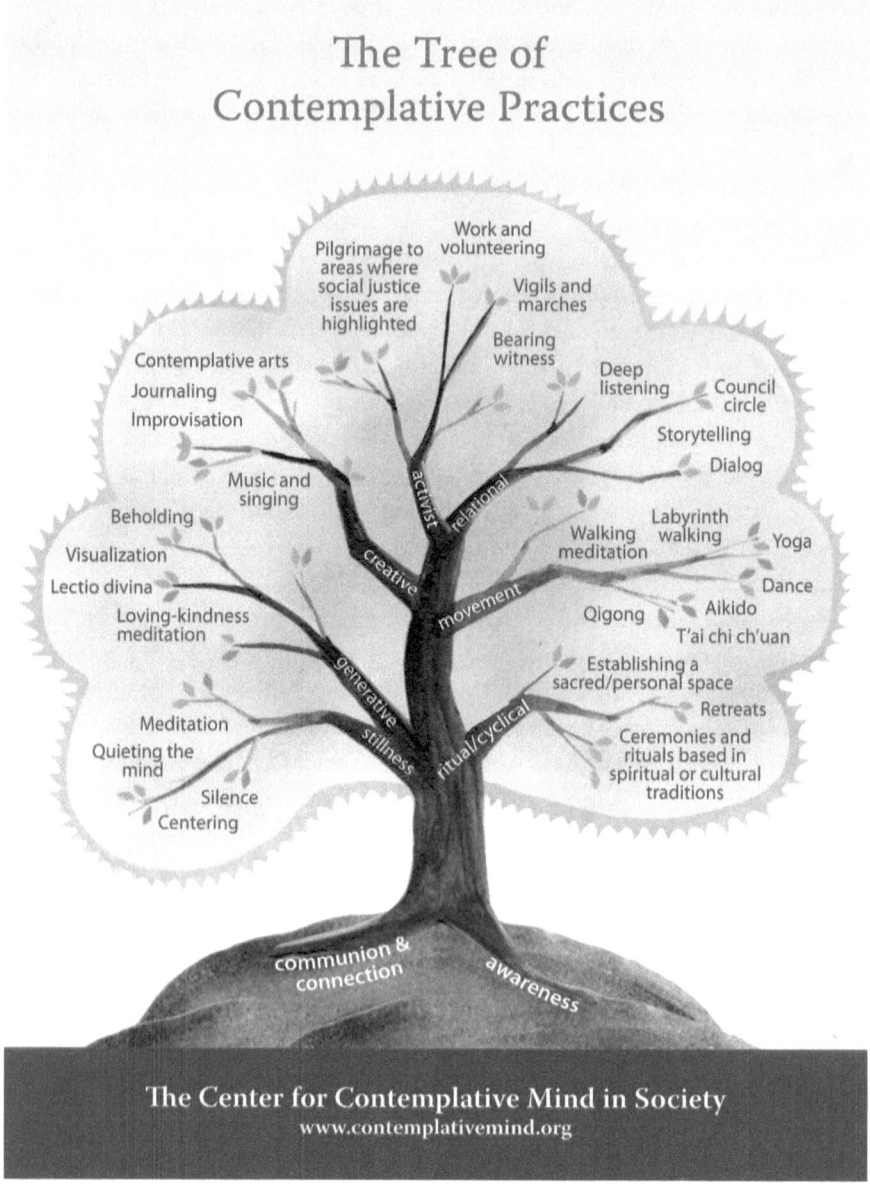

Figure 1. The Tree of Contemplative Practices.
The Center for Contemplative Mind in Society, 2012. Used by permission.

Fellow contemplative educator, O'Reilley, warns of the importance of both finding inspiration from others using contemplative methods in their courses while also staying true to our motivations for incorporating those methods in our classrooms in the first place. In her book on using Buddhism and Quakerism in her writing and literature classrooms, O'Reilley cautions us that "when we talk about teaching within a contemplative frame of reference, I think we should keep our prescriptions to a minimum. I want to sketch the lines of a certain approach, but I don't want to trespass into another teacher's prayer hall" (1998, p. 14). I proceed in much the same way here, using this book to document how I have created contemplative spaces in my writing classes inspired by my personal practice of yoga and the ways I have begun to see yoga and writing as complementary creative endeavors. And while I could choose any modern practice of yoga, I've chosen Iyengar because it is what I practice and because it is highly adaptable, as I note in my preface, though this style is also arguably the most influential school of modern yoga (DeMichelis, 2005, p. 15). I invite my readers to find their own "prayer halls."

In concentrating my efforts around yoga, I am echoing the calls within Judith Beth Cohen's and Geraldine DeLuca's recent articles, The Missing Body—Yoga and Higher Education and Headstands, Writing and the Rhetoric of Self-Acceptance, respectively, to actively seek out the connections between writing pedagogy and yoga practice. Cohen argues that the most obvious connection between the two is the focus on process and movement, and DeLuca inhabits this fluid process in her article as she documents the difficulty of accepting her limitations as a yoga student and discovers a parallelism in this humbling exercise that she can draw upon as a writing teacher. Through her struggling practice of headstand, *sirsasana* in Sanskirt, DeLuca learns the pedagogical value of "radical self-acceptance," or of accepting where she is in the present moment instead of trying to push away the parts of her reality she'd rather not face. In doing so, she challenges the commonplace that forward motion is the only way growth in our writing and teaching of writing can be measured.

Like critical thinking, mindfulness is a particular, intentional application of awareness and is best seen as a skill that can be developed with practice. As a yogi, I practice mindfulness each time I sit on my mat to mediate and each time I flow through a series of poses, a *vinyasana*, linking breath and movement together. It is this sense of mindfulness I hoped the students in my preface were exposed to as they experienced moving their bodies through poses. But, mindfulness doesn't just stay on the mat; not only can mindfulness learned through contemplative traditions transfer to our daily activities such as writing, but the very act of performing our day-to-day experiences can become a viable means of practicing mindfulness and learning to develop contemplative presence. Thus, the act of teaching can itself become a contemplative practice when driven by mindfulness, and our most mundane classroom routines (such as taking roll or pausing for reflection) can become contemplative exercises in themselves (by using this time to have students sit in a moment of silence).

It is in this spirit of self-acceptance for where I am in the present moment that I offer this book as an initial exploration of how a feminist writing pedagogue who is also a committed yogi might take yoga into the writing classroom and make sense of what happens in both practical and theoretical terms. My comprehensive goal is to see what feminist theory, writing studies and contemplative practice have to offer each other, and how we might build responsible incarnations of contemplative pedagogy in their generative coupling. This is important work as the field investigates how crucial metacognition is to students' ability to learn and transfer writing skills and processes. Yoga offers mindfulness as the "meta" link that bridges learning, self-reflection and movement. While my investigation will at times take me to the practical and at other moments to the theoretical, it is grounded firmly in the lessons of my embodied experience on the mat and in the classroom. Like O'Reilley, I "[l]et methodology follow from the particular" (1998, p. 14) in my application of contemplative writing pedagogy.

I noticed early on in my own training that both yogis and compositionists share a fundamental premise about the importance of lived theory: as a master of yoga has put it, "your practice is your laboratory" (Iyengar, 2005, p. 102). This humble attitude means that contemplative educators must be willing to show their vulnerability as learners in the classroom, alongside their students. As a colleague recently said in response to a conference presentation of mine on contemplative pedagogy, the most radical element of this kind of teaching is the way it positions teachers as students too and asks them to engage directly in the learning experiences of their classrooms, destabilizing their complete authority in the classroom. Like others before me, I am not a certified yoga teacher, but I still teach my students basic poses and breathing exercises. Indeed, I have found that approaching these activities as a learner too helps to shift the power dynamics in my classrooms in productive ways. And, while I've had the very good fortune of bringing in my yoga teachers to help expose my writing students to contemplative practice, this is not a necessary element of contemplative pedagogy. Despite a handful of visits each semester from these yoga teachers, I remain the primary resource for students since we practice every class meeting. For readers contemplating using contemplative practice in their own classrooms, though, I do encourage reaching out to local contemplative communities to find support. I never expected to find yoga instructors willing to teach my students for nothing but a cup of coffee and a few conversations in return—at not just one but at the two universities I taught during the drafting of this book—but I did. Contemplative communities are full of giving and generous people, as my experience highlights.

In sum, there are many ways to integrate contemplation, silence and focused movement into our classes, and contemplative pedagogy can support all of these ways. What distinguishes contemplative pedagogies is their attention to the body as a primary site for mindful reflection, contemplative awareness and centeredness—not the practice of yoga. Just as a voice teacher might instruct students on deep belly breathing or a drama teacher might get students moving around, we too can teach students mindful breathing and movement to help them work through writing anxiety and show them stretches to help them generate new ideas. The goal of contemplative pedagogy is not to turn students into martial artists or yogis; rather, it is to show them what they can learn by paying attention to their bodies.

PRACTICING THEORY

Just as my writing classroom is the locus of invention for my teaching theory, my own yoga practice was the first research space for this project. While I've followed a home practice of yoga for years, it was only more recently that I began to explore the connections between yoga and writing—and only because they kept colliding in ways I could no longer ignore. Knowing how centered and calm I felt after practicing yoga, I found myself naturally creating a writing routine that integrated yoga breaks. As often as my schedule would allow, I'd wake up early to write and when I felt my attention wander, I would break for time on my mat. Initially, these breaks were simply geared to get me away from the computer and were taken more with the intent to develop my *sadhana* or practice of yoga than to sustain my writing. Even so, after these breaks, I felt revived and ... something more. I began to see that "something more" as a sense of mindfulness and clarity cultivated through my *yogasana* practice that transferred into my proceeding writing sessions. These were different breaks than those I took to watch television, take a nap or fold laundry; none of those acts felt like a continuation of the writing process the way that yoga did. Yoga, true to its promise to cultivate mindfulness that transfers off the mat, was helping me grow a deep awareness I could feel seeping into my writing. Of course, this awareness remained only as strong as I was; my motivation to write still threw a fence around my attentiveness.

It only seemed natural to begin integrating more yoga into my long writing sessions, leaving my mat open near my computer in order to isolate poses as needed, such as stretching my rounded "computer" shoulders with *gomukhasana* arms, hooking the hands together near the shoulder blades by sending one arm up to the sky and down the body and the other around the back body to reach up and meet the first. I didn't see this practice in line with the commercially-popular "office yoga," which is stretching for its own sake, but as part of a writing process that worked with the body and respected its effect on making meaning as much as that of the mind. When my body was tense and tired, I was less likely to read my sources compassionately and more likely to skim them for points of weakness without listening to their arguments. As my body self-awareness grew through a combined practice, I gradually came to see yoga not as a miracle cure to all of what ails writers, but as a helpful tool for us to transform our mental and physical writing habits and rituals.

The metaphoric and the literal began to bleed together through my integrated practice and made me begin to question the value for writers of not just practicing yoga but also understanding the philosophies behind such contemplative practices. I was drawn to the metaphoric connections between the practice of writing and the practice of yoga; they suddenly screamed for my attention. Yoga, both as a philosophy and as a tradition of movement and breath awareness, is highly literary and symbolic. Literal balance developed in *asanas* or poses is thought to translate to a metaphoric balance in the yogi's life. In tree pose, for instance, you learn to find balance in the constant sway of your body by developing a mind-body awareness and strength that works *with* such movement in order not to dominate but to channel the sway productively. Tree pose literally trains the body to find balance, and this is understood to transfer off the sticky mat and to give the yogi poise and balance amidst the undulations of life. Nothing ever simply stays on the mat. The body is the hinge for such lessons so that when we learn to work with it, we grow and advance in all aspects of our lives. Yoga's core focus on balance, flexibility, consciousness, non-violence and awareness was intimately familiar since these were qualities I recognized in good writing and as possessed by strong, feminist writers. These were qualities I could appreciate in both forms of self-expression before I ever began to write my way through them. I'd taught Rogerian argument in my writing classes as a means of encouraging students to question our society's "argument culture," as Deborah Tannen (1998) calls it, for instance, and I'd long admired disability studies writer Nancy Mairs for her pithy and often humorous reminders to become aware of our writing bodies.

At the same time that I was exploring the union of yoga and writing, I came into contact with Jeffery Davis' *The Journey from the Center to the Page* (2004), which advocates infusing yoga practice into the creative writing process. Davis' intent to use yoga to get writers to work with and through the physical body and its experiences resonated with me even if his call for "authenticity" and his concentration on fiction writing did not. In the end, his book serves more as an inspiration for what I describe here rather than a source. As my own sustained practice of yoga converged with the process of my burgeoning academic research on embodiment and writing, I saw how yoga provided not only a new lens for my work but also a set of practices I could use to bring the body into the domain of the writing classroom, hopefully teaching students to think about their bodies as generators of meaning. This contemplative goal has consequences for feminist pedagogy.

BRINGING TOGETHER THE FEMINIST AND THE CONTEMPLATIVE

My practice of yoga has been a space for me to enact my feminism. Through yoga, I continue to learn acceptance of my body while not reducing myself to it. When I read the *Yoga Sutras* and stumble across passages about moving toward self-understanding and enlightenment through union of the body, heart and mind, I am struck by the congruence between these goals and feminisms' focus on egalitarianism and experience as the means by which change and understanding occurs (the personal is always political). And so my thinking about contemplative pedagogy is filtered through my feminism and, indeed, strengthened by it. In turn, I use this book to explore not only the theory and practice of embracing contemplative pedagogy in the writing classroom but also to explore what happens when we consciously approach this pedagogy as feminist. Yoga can be seen as a feminist's guilty pleasure, a time when she submits to our society's obsessive regulations of women's bodies to be tight and toned, and feeds the capitalist-patriarchal system by purchasing hundred-dollar Lululemon (lululemon athletica®) yoga pants because they make her backside look good. What this characterization points to is the problematic ways that yoga has been commercialized and gendered in American society and not necessarily an intolerance for feminism at yoga's core.

Yoga's commercialization has sometimes reduced this contemplative practice to a form of exercise, and a hypersexualized one at that. This hasn't gone unnoticed by the most committed of yogis. A popular journal for practitioners, *Yoga Journal*, recently published a letter written by the publication's co-founder which condemned the magazine's ads for their use of almost- or completely-naked models to sell products ranging from yoga clothes to yoga mats. If modern incarnations of yoga reveal capitalist misogyny, and classic yoga texts like the *Yoga Sutras* are immersed in Eastern patriarchy, then what makes yoga—or contemplative philosophy and practice altogether—useful for feminist inquiry?

While I recognize the important historical and cultural complications raised by this line of questioning, my use of Iyengar yoga and yoga philosophy as a mainstay for my pedagogy's implication in the contemplative takes a hopeful view of its usefulness for feminist writing pedagogies. While I do recognize that ancient yogic texts are steeped in the traditions of patriarchy and that some modern Western applications still reflect these traditions as well as our own, I believe there are just as many congruencies between yoga and feminism ripe for consideration, such as a commitment to change through transformation as well as a spirit of equanimity that eschews binaries. While the task of delineating the ways in which yoga philosophy is reflective of the patriarchies in which it is practiced is worthwhile, that is not my aim here. Rather, I am engaged in understanding how yoga can sustain the kind of feminist, embodied-contemplative inquiry I am after.

Feminist studies is uniquely situated in the university as interdisciplinary. This refusal to sit still and play nice when it comes to matters of academic institutionalism is a feature it shares with contemplative pedagogy, which has sprung up in departments as diverse as biology and religion. I use this interdisciplinarity to my advantage. A key figure for me is scientist-theorist Donna Haraway who provides a means to reclaim our writing bodies as lived, fleshy presences—the kind around which Tompkins creates personal vignettes—while avoiding essentialist criticism that tends to follow claims to the organic body. Because Haraway speaks from the point of view as a scientist, she is interested in models of subjectivity that better reflect our lived realities as biological beings living as part of and among a material world; and because she too writes from her perspective as a feminist theorist, she wants models that do not eschew the theoretical progress we have made in the name of postmodernism, which has helped us understand the social construction of many of our "givens." Instead of seeking any sort of definitive answers by drawing new lines between nature and culture, Haraway finds promise in the indeterminacy of materiality and the way respect for our flesh necessitates a stance of openness as opposed to the false closure of other postmodern variations of the subject, which tend to espouse a thinly-veiled linguistic determinism. Haraway's alternative epistemology consequently offers an alternative to the etheralization of the body that Howson targets by leaving the organic body as a source of necessary tension to keep our theorizing in check—a tension too often lost. As a result, she mediates contemplative pedagogies' focus on the center and poststructualist decentering by insisting on the generative paradox of embracing both simultaneously. Simply, she helps me to theorize the writer within a field of "commonsense materiality" (Sanchez, 2012, p. 235) while remaining sensitive to the rhetorical acts that situate this writer also within a field of discourse. While feminists writing today have sometimes leapfrogged over her in attempt to embrace newer theorists, Haraway, I believe, leads the way in our journey to rethink the body materially and in a spirit true to contemplative practice.

Haraway doesn't just address our dangerous tendency to efface materiality; she pins hope on the body for revamping our systems of meaning-making and epistemologies in order to bring about real change in the world, converging her project with the central foci of writing studies *and* contemplative practice. What's more, she corrects those who claim the body without asserting its agency by insisting that we need to be concerned not only with the materiality of subject formation but also with the agentive status of bodies themselves—bodies that shape language *as much as* language shapes them. It's not just that the body is involved in our meaning-making processes, but that it conditions our systems of knowledge from the very start. This is consistent with contemplative pedagogies' reliance on the physical body as the primary structure for self-realization. With Haraway, I will theorize a feminist-minded "writing yogi" for contemplative pedagogies, a mode of authorship that agentizes student writing and validates students' experiences of embodiment. My notion of writing yogis insists on a level of conscious awareness of our writing bodies; we certainly always write as bodies, but few of us are ready to claim them—especially in academic environments beholden to disembodiment. Further, a focus on writing yogis within this book indicates a concern with how writers *experience* their embodiment and *practice* it rather than on a semiotics of material placement, even if situatedness will be a key term to define this experience. The writing yogi is a concept that I play off of in my project's title, and one I will further flesh out in the following chapters.

Writing yogis is an appropriate marker because contemplative pedagogy both re-theorizes the writing subject as writing body-heart-mind and actualizes this theory by engaging writers in contemplative acts that move their whole beings. Such pedagogies are important to writing studies because they encourage mindfulness of writing and learning processes in ways that promote the academic work accomplished in our classes while at the same time remaining committed to a larger scope of a writer's physical and emotional well-being. What further marks these pedagogies is their combined focus on self-examination and awareness of our connectedness with others as complementary understandings that can be deepened by the learning process. In a widely-cited article on contemplative education, Tobin Hart claims that contemplative knowing rests on opening the "contemplative mind" which is "activated through a wide range of approaches—from poetry to meditation—that are designed to quiet and shift the habitual chatter of the mind to cultivate the capacity of deepened awareness, concentration, and insight" (2004, p. 29). Once the mind is opened in such ways to create inner awareness, a "corresponding opening occurs toward the world around us" (2004, p. 29). While I can't take his term as my own since it advances the misnomer that contemplation is solely a practice of the mind, Hart's understandings rearticulate what it means to be focused on a "whole life" pedagogy and show how a developed sense of embodied interiority necessitates an equal connection to exteriority and to others. Mindful knowing is, by default, connected knowing as it refuses the mindless fragmentation of our scattered lives. Along the way, this contemplative model may help student writers find balance and compassion on and off the page; teaching difference as embodied may lead to stronger and more pragmatic understandings of social justice and personal transformation through the formation of an embodied, feminist-contemplative ethics.

YOUR BODY IS YOUR MUSE:
THE EMBODIED IMAGINATION IN YOGA

And so I arrive full-circle back to my opening narrative in this introduction. My struggle in downward-facing dog highlights the potential value of yoga's insights for the writing classroom and provides the thread that ties together the braid of this book's chapters and interchapters. Namely, my difficulties in downward-facing dog attest to the ways yoga asks its practitioners to be embodied imaginers, realizing meaning with and through our feeling flesh, against modern impulses that deny the intelligence of the body. If I hope to improve my practice of *Adho Mukha Svanasana*, I have to learn to use my body awareness to *feel* my way toward full expression of my *asanas*. This requires me to lay aside my academic neurosis of attempting to control, ignore or transcend my body for the sake of identifying myself solely with my mind. It's not that I must define myself as *only* body, but that I must begin to imagine myself as an interrelated whole, not in parts, in order to grow intellectually, spiritually[3] and physically.

My practice of poses like downward-dog teaches me that verbal abstractions in the form of the directions my yoga teacher gives to her students must pair with our actual experiences of them. For instance, Holly's frequent injunction to push the front knee into the back knee in down-dog means nothing to me unless

I can both imagine this process and make real these imaginings though practiced embodiment and self-awareness. In my struggle recounted at the beginning of this introduction, I knew where, in theory, my body should be placed for successful execution of the pose, but I couldn't connect this with my practice because I assumed that the theory was what mattered most. But, as I have learned, it is only with awareness of my organic body and my physical and emotional feelings can I be "in" the pose as opposed to simply forcing myself through its actions.

Moving from the mat to the classroom, I correspondingly define the embodied imagination as the faculty by which body, heart and mind work together to bring meaning and understanding to writing under the praxis of contemplative pedagogy. Imagining, as I see it through a feminist and yogic lens, is integrative, thoughtful and emotive. Its axis is the heart; what is felt both physiologically and psychically shapes the interrelationship between the body and the mind. I recognize the ways imagining is often limited to describing fantastical or illusory mental processes, flights of fancy. But, following feminist usage and the yogic philosophies of Iyengar, founder of the yoga method that I practice, I hope to extend the concept of the imagination to talk about the creative fusion of the intelligent, organic body and mind toward the construction of present realities and future possibilities in writing. These realities and possibilities are based on the knowledge we construct from our experiences (what we understand) and our affective positions toward other bodies as a result of these experiences (how we feel). The imagining process is therefore a situated and recursive one that involves our bodies and minds. Put differently, our imaginings always occur in the context of our material environments and within the frame of our flesh; similarly, our bodies must embrace and enact the dreams and ideas of our intellect for them to *mean* and to be acted upon. As bell hooks puts it in the opening quotation of my epigraph, what we imagine helps to create our reality, which shapes what we believe to be imaginable from the start. In the embrace of imagination, the body interprets and structures our ideas, lending validity to the idea that responsible imaginings are those that remain accountable to our flesh.

The embodied imagination provides a new method of inquiry in composition studies, one that takes its lineage from feminism and an Eastern tradition of Iyengar yoga that challenges hierarchical dualities and seeks integration and mindfulness at its core. In their recent *College Composition and Communication* article, Gesa E. Kirsch and Jacqueline J. Royster trace contemporary feminist usage of what they coin the "critical imagination" which becomes one of the three "terms of engagement" they trace throughout their historical survey of feminist rhetorical practices (2010, p. 648). Working alongside "strategic contemplation" and "social circulation," the critical imagination is a strategy of inquiry or a tool "to engage, as it were, in hypothesizing ... as a means for searching methodically, not so much for immutable truth, but instead for what is likely or possible, given the facts in hand" (Kirsch & Royster, 2010, p. 650). A look at Royster's earlier *Traces of a Stream* gives a fuller picture of their concept.

In her book, Royster develops this conception of the imagination in order to propose how feminist reconstruction might aid in the making of historical narratives about ancestral African women's history. Within the historical narrative, the

> imagination becomes a critical skill, that is, the ability to see the possibility of certain experiences even if we cannot know the specificity of them .... So defined, imagination functions as a critical skill in questioning a viewpoint, an experience, an event, and so on, and in remaking interpretative frameworks based on that questioning. (2000, p. 83)

The imagination so defined enables conversation and interaction between the feminist researcher and her subjects, according to Kirsch and Royster, as it connects the past and present with future "vision[s] of hope" (2010, p. 652-53). Because it is grounded in the particularities of experience, the critical imagination helps facilitate an embodied practice that focuses on research as a lived process (2010, p. 657).

In another permutation, feminists Nira Yuval-Davis and Marcel Stoetzler have claimed the "situated imagination" as necessary to the workings of transversal politics, which seeks to dialogue through difference without overwriting it (2002, p.316). Yuval-Davis credits feminists in Bologna, Italy for the cultivation of this democratic, feminist political practice based on three interlocking concepts: standpoint theory's reminder that because differing viewpoints produce varying bodies of knowledge, any one body of knowledge is essentially unfinished; that even those who are positioned similarly may not share the same values or identifications; and that notions of equality need not be replaced by respect for difference but can be used to encompass difference (Yuval-Davis, 1999, pp. 1-2). As I will in Chapter Two, Yuval-Davis uses Haraway's notion of situatedness, which is multiple and embodied, to underscore the importance of differential positioning in knowledge-making practices. She and her co-author introduce the situated imagination as a conceptual tool that works in tandem with situated knowledge in feminist epistemology.

Working at the intersections of present reality and future hope for change, the situated imagination shapes experience into knowledge by helping to construct meaning as well as to stretch it in new directions. Even if situated like knowledge, the imagination, which is both self- and other-directed, can help to establish common ground, especially important to transversal politics (Yuval-Davis & Stoetzler, 2002, p. 316). Imagining is understood within Yuval-Davis' project to be both a social faculty as well as a bodily one, or a "gateway to the body, on the one hand, and society, on the other hand" (Yuval-Davis & Stoetzler, 2002, p. 325). Imagining and thinking aren't just bridged in the process of understanding, however, they are inseparable and contingent on each other so that, as both authors note, "intellect and imagination, these terms do not refer to clearly separate faculties or 'spheres,' but merely to dialogical moments in a multidimensional mental process" (Yuval-Davis & Stoetzler, 2002, p. 326). The circularity is key. I take this as a reminder of the companionate nature of thinking and imagining which converge in the physical body to create knowledge as well as hope.

For my conception of the embodied imagination, I chose to stitch the best together from this quilt of feminist definitions. What I like about Kirsch and Royster's critical imagination is its focus on the *skill* of imagining; what this means for our writing classrooms is that we can teach students to deepen their imaginative embrace when constructing new ideas, filtering through their own experiences or when presented with others' experiences or ideas. The embodied imagination I propose resembles the critical imagination in that it too works as a method of inquiry that allows us to imagine creatively that which initially may not be a reality, that which may yet be eclipsed by our personal experience or that which we would like to change, remake or revise. But, I don't accept the critical imagination as my own because I find it engages too weak a model of embodiment, even if it does acknowledge materiality in the process of researching, reminding us of the personal bodies who investigate as well as the particular bodies studied. And partly because I do not come at my project from a historicist perspective, I find it too limiting to talk mostly about the imagination as a frame for possibility and not also as participating in a concrete reality; I wish for a less speculative application of the imagination. Yuval-Davis and Stoetzler provide an earthier or more rooted definition for my tastes, and it is happy coincidence that they too draw from Haraway's theories, connecting, to an extent, our projects. But while Yuval-Davis and Stoetzler divide their episteme into two functions, that of imagining and knowing, I feel this is a restrictive model that eclipses the role feeling has to play in meaning-making. Consequently, I concentrate on three related processes brought together under the rubric of embodiment and representative of the contemplative: imagining, thinking and feeling.

The embodied imagination, as such, can be understood as a space for negotiation between situated thinking and situated feeling toward new possibilities and a mindful awareness of the present (and, therein, the future). Thinking of the imagination as the spider that spins the sticky web that helps connect our feelings and thoughts to fashion such awareness coincides with yet another feminist forwarding of this facility: Haraway's definition of the imagination as the connective tissue between feminist networks of meaning wherein individuals are not simply involved in critiquing or distancing, but are interested in establishing coalitional epistemologies and methodologies to bring people together. Haraway claims she "hates" the model of negative criticality that only sees value in dismantling arguments so that you don't have to implicate yourself in the struggle, "rooted in the fear of embracing something with all its messiness and dirtiness and imperfection" (Haraway & Goodeve, 2000, pp. 111-112). Of course, the body stands as a living symbol of the "messiness" we have often locked out in fear of losing the certainty of closure. Working from a place of connection, Haraway is not simply involved in critiquing but is "involved in building alternative ontologies, specifically via the use of the imaginative" (Haraway & Goodeve, 2000, p. 120). Feminist contemplative pedagogies provide such an alternative.

Also working within a framework of connection, I will be less interested in delineating the lines between the organic body and the cultural body (or, incidentally, feelings as biological or social) and more interested in a holistic approach that respects the companionate nature of the body as both marked and marking. Haraway explains to her interviewer in *How Like a Leaf* that defining her methods as part of a "worldly practice" as opposed to aligning them with either side of the inherently problematic nature/ culture dichotomy emphasizes the "imploded set of things where the physiology of one's body, the coursing of blood and hormones and the operations of chemicals—the fleshiness of the organism—intermesh with the whole life of the organism" (Haraway & Goodeve, 2000, p. 110). In the same way, contemplative writing can help form a "worldly," "whole life" pedagogy that takes into account the ecological connections between the body and mind, nature and culture, rationality and emotion which we tend to elide for the relative simplicity of academic processes of inquiry. Owing more to Aristotelian logic than inquiry vested in awareness of the contemplative connections between body, heart and mind, traditional processes of academic inquiry focused on objectivism have excluded and/ or marginalized alternative ways of knowing such as contemplative and connected knowing. As these typical processes are driven by narrow applications of problem solving through logic, they tend toward closure via disconnection and skepticism as opposed to the open-endedness of the imagination.

When inquiry *is* driven by the imagination, we end up with projects of connected knowing, or the process of understanding difference through connection, not distance. In contrast to separate knowers who experience the self as autonomous, connected knowers experience the self in relational webs (Belenky, Clinchy, Goldberger, & Tarule, 1973, pp. 113-123). If the primary action of separate knowing is that of breaking down, connected knowing is characterized by building both on and anew. Likewise, we can see the process of embodied imagining as connected; to genuinely connect, we need to be aware of our thoughts and feelings and attend to others' whether real or anticipated. In these ways, we can extend positioning not only as the key for grounding knowledge claims but also our imaginings. When we focus on the imagination, we change discussions of inquiry from finding *the* answer to a problem to investigating multiple possibilities *and* testing these alternatives against our embodied realities, lending more weight toward embodied pragmatism than a transcendent critical analysis that ignores our corporeality. In other words, the embodied imagination becomes a tool of mindfulness for feminist pedagogies. As we imagine, we slow down and pay attention; we reflect and notice; we connect and draw together.

In the afterword to *The Teacher's Body,* Madeleine Grumet notes that the "body throws a horizon around [the] imagination … it tethers [the] imagination to a set of possibilities which, although they are protean, are not limitless" (2003, p. 274). Yuval-Davis and Stoetzler say much the same: "Imagination is situated; our imaginary horizons are affected by the positioning of our gaze" (2002, p. 327). How we imagine ourselves and our world matters because it shapes the meaning we take from our experiences and the receptiveness with which we approach others' realities. Imagining ourselves as situated, embodied beings accords respect for differential positioning and compels us to respect the very real consequences of our materiality in our worlds and in our words. Connected to the body and attentive to difference, these feminist versions of the imagination are a far cry from the neo-Romantic "creative imagination" of expressivism.

Yoga philosophy can be seen to build on Grument's idea that the body serves as an anchor for the imagination. Yoga is also a contemplative practice that actualizes the mindfulness at the heart of the embodied imagination. Iyengar's thoughts on the imagination are the second wellspring for my concept because they stress the application of the imagination in our ordinary lives as we bring our imaginings to bear on our realities in order to shape and to change them. Iyengar explains that the imagination must be steadily applied to our reality. Comparing this application to the writing process, he notes, "[a] writer may dream of the plot for a new novel, but unless he applies himself to pen and paper, his ideas have no value …. Never mind the idea, write it down"(2005, p. 156). The embodied imagination described here is the fire that transforms the writer's thoughts into reality on the page and in her life, differentiating imagining from daydreaming;

the latter of the two lacks the pragmatic pulse. *Asana*, or practice of the physical poses of yoga, is the link that trains us to bring our thoughts to bear on our realities: "[a]sana practice brings mind and body into harmony for this task …. The coordination between them that we learn in asana will enable us to turn the shape of our visions into the substance of our lives" (Iyengar, 2005, p. 157). *Asana* teaches us to claim our materiality by developing our physical and imaginative faculties. This is not just about imagining possibility then, but using the imagination as a source of intentional doing. Just as in writing, it is the process that becomes the focus.

Asana teaches us to embody our imaginings by bringing together the intelligence of the body, which "is a fact … is real" and the intelligence of the brain which "is only imagination" (Iyengar, 2005, p. 63). "The imagination has to be made real. The brain may dream of doing a difficult backbend today, but it cannot force the impossible even on to a willing body. We are always trying to progress, but inner cooperation is essential" (Iyengar, 2005, p. 63). To return once more to my own practice as an example, I must make my imaginings of *Adho Mukha Svanasana* "real," or embodied, by listening to my body and tapping into my feelings through continued practice of the pose. This means I can't simply overwrite by body's intelligence, which grounds my intellect: "the brain may say: 'We can do it.' But the knee says: 'Who are you to dictate to me? It is for me to say whether I can do it or not'" (Iyengar, 2005, p. 30). It means that I must begin to imagine myself as not just consciousness or body but both by interweaving brain and body into intelligent movement that respects the limits of my present practice while stretching toward a future of what may be. The greater my personal awareness in the pose and the more experiential knowledge I gather, the more possibility my current and future pose holds. This reality rests in my present actions so that my imaginings are embodied through the fruits of my labor. That is, embodied imaginers develop awareness of habits by tapping into the intelligence of our cells so that we are able to challenge old patterns of doing and entrenched beliefs by *being in the present moment*, for it is the actions of today that will bring about the growth of tomorrow.

To be present, we must be flexible and must respect the fluidity with which we interact with others, be they subjects or objects, in the world. I will capitalize on this literal-metaphoric flexibility in Chapter Three. Gloria Anzaldua is an example of an author who embodies this sort of flexibility and awareness in her writings. It is for this reason that I often use her as a resource in my writing classes. In *Borderlands,* she argues that while "we are taught that the body is an ignorant animal; intelligence dwells only in the head," "the body is smart. It does not discern between external stimuli and stimuli from the imagination. It reacts equally viscerally to events from the imagination as it does to 'real' events" (1999, pp. 59-60). With the congruence between her thoughts and those I have just explored from Iyengar, it is no surprise that Anzaldua adopts the concept of "yoga of the body" in a 1983 interview to explain the ways a writer's creativity is filtered through the body and how readers respond to this viscerally (2000, p. 77). This author's essay in *Borderlands*, *Tilli, Tlapalli*: The Path of the Red and Black Ink, dramatizes the process of writing from the body and with the body while viewing the text produced as taking on a fleshy presence itself. About the visceral reaction of reading and its connection to a yoga of the body, Anzaldua reminds us after reflecting upon the 1983 interview years later that

> [e]very word you read hits you physiologically—your blood pressure changes; your cells; your bones, your muscle [stet] are moved by a beautiful poem, a tragic episode. So that's the kind of yoga that I want: a yoga filtered through the body and through the imagination, the emotions, the spirit, and the soul. (2000, p. 77)

Over thirty years ago, Anzaldua started a conversation about yoga, writing and the imagination that I want to continue here within the frame of composition studies and contemplative writing pedagogies.

A FEW NOTES ON STRUCTURE AND CONTENT

As indicated above, this project is invested in a faithfulness of being within a "worldly" pedagogy that concentrates on the non-duality of experience. To respect the united aspects of being, I have yoked mind, body and heart together. This structure unlocks the power of contemplative learning as applied to writing pedagogies: such pedagogies are transformative of the writer's whole being in an ethical and relational context which takes matter as the connective substance that facilitates a developed self- and other-awareness.

A true praxis, the theory and practice of yoga reciprocally inform one another. To highlight the strength of contemplative connectedness where the imaginative becoming of theory feeds and is fed by the lived practice of being, I have followed each of my three theoretical chapters on body, heart and mind with a corresponding "interchapter," an equally-long section that reports on my efforts to practice contemplative writing pedagogy in the classroom and analyzes students' reactions to it. In doing so, these sections speak back to my chapters and showcase the pedagogical interventions and applications of the theory covered in them.

The interchapters also loosely apply and yet purposefully confuse the chapter's divisions between body, heart and mind, reminding us that while writing may be rooted in the linear, our embodied identities are most certainly not. Overall, the chapter-interchapter structure of my project supports my combined focus on theory and practice, dialoguing lived research from qualitative case studies with the theories from yoga, feminism and composition studies explored in my chapters in order to "speak back" to the theory. The interplay between chapters and interchapters testifies to my belief in the power of teaching practice to generatively complicate, shape and transform pedagogical theories—just as the lived experience of *being* a body in the world can inform our theories of embodiment.

Chapter One responds to the recent call for "different" theory that recognizes the writer's commonsense materiality. I trace the steps feminists have already made to embrace the organic body, journeying from Tompkins and Hindman to Fleckenstein and others, and introduce contemplative writing as a viable theoretical and pedagogical approach. I offer a contemplative view of the writer as a "writing yogi" and address the need for this moniker by examining three main tenants of embodiment from yoga: that our flesh is intelligent because our consciousness is diffused throughout the body and not simply located in the brain; that embodiment is uniquely experienced and situated; even if it is also the case that because of our shared material nature, the yogi's inner turn to the center is simultaneously an unfolding to the external. I dialogue these three core understandings with Haraway's theories of embodiment. The dialogue allows me to enact the self-reflexivity that is key to contemplative pedagogical approaches and to insist that contemplative pedagogies can be strengthened by feminism's overt attention to what happens when we view the body as an anchor and tool of our self- and other-awareness.

The first interchapter then shares details of how teachers might help students see themselves as writing yogis. I focus on how I primed my students to be receptive to an integrated yoga-writing practice within my application of feminist contemplative pedagogy. In this section, I detail a composite account from a string of recent first-year writing courses[4] that asked students to investigate the corporeality of the writing process by examining writing habits and rituals. The language of habits and rituals is one that provides students a feminist, embodied hermeneutic by which to re-evaluate their processes. This is language my students cultivated through a beginning assignment that required them to complete a multi-step, self-ethnographic study of their writing. As it gave students a fresh perspective on writing and engaged them in a metacognitive analysis of their process, this assignment unearthed questions of the body's impact on writing and highlighted the transformative potential of yoga.

Introduction

As with my other interchapters, while I draw from the theoretical framing provided by the chapter that precedes this section, I concentrate my efforts on the practical dynamics of the assignment itself and focus, in particular, on student writing. Allowing students to speak through their writing in this section reiterates the claim I make repeatedly about the respect afforded to individual bodies in feminist contemplative pedagogy. And as with all student writing and reactions in this book, my accounts are drawn from a series of first-year writing classes and do not reflect a single class. Because I moved institutional homes in the process of researching and writing this book, the first-year classrooms represented in my composite course represent a wide sample of students. While my methods are primarily qualitative in nature, my sample includes students from both an East-coast private, liberal arts school and a Mid-Atlantic public liberal arts university. While my course content morphed some over the years I taught the first-year composition courses represented here, the general pedagogical approach remained consistent.

Having explored the cost of ignoring the writing body and addressed the benefits of situating the body at the center of our theories and classroom practices of writing, I use Chapter Two to highlight what feminist contemplative pedagogy expands our learning approaches to include and what effects this has on the writing yogi. I review the ways body criticism in composition studies has been stunted by the conflation of the body with the personal—even advocates of the body such as Hindman have fallen prey to this slippage. A contemplative understanding of presence, I argue there, is far less embedded in the tropes of the theoretical body, and forwards instead a lived, moment-to-moment understanding of materiality. Presence allows us to approach a writer's agency as singular, situated in a particular body, and located via her interaction with other material bodies—even if it is also social. Finally, I explore how situated knowledge calls for this kind of presence as situated knowers refuse to ignore embodied particularities in the quest of understanding themselves and the world.

Interchapter Two investigates the situated knowledge students develop in a contemplative writing classroom about the writing process itself. I use the recently released and popular Framework for Success in Postsecondary Writing to explore how writers develop successful habits of mind by engaging in an integrated yoga-writing practice driven by mindfulness. Drawing on preceding chapters' discussions of mindfulness as an embodied process of metacognition that involves writers in an analysis of how they and others experience and practice embodiment, I illustrate how writing yogis approach learning and writing purposefully and responsibly. I focus on my students' execution of three of the Framework's eight habits: openness, persistence and metacognition. Examining student writing for these representative skills, I argue that contemplative pedagogies can foster the habits set forth in the Framework, goals we as a field have established as intentions for our instructional practice. I show how a contemplative approach to the writing process helps students develop the habits forwarded by the Framework and also uses means that develop them as habits of mind *and* body, penetrating students' lives at a deeper level and giving them a foundation for approaching their educations contemplatively and their writing mindfully.

In the third chapter, I argue that because mindfulness practices like yoga teach writers to exchange mindless rumination on and judgment of experiences for open awareness, writers who engage in these practices learn to better monitor and understand their thoughts and feelings. Feminist theory within (Lynn Worsham, Laura Micciche) and outside our disciplinary bounds (Sarah Jaggar, Haraway, Sara Amhed) creates an exigency for the visibility of emotion within contemplative writing pedagogy and anchors my investigation of how we might enable students to become passionate, embodied imaginers, constructively engaging their emotions instead of simply managing or dismissing them. Yoga teaches writers to mindfully approach feeling as an agentive force of the body; it also offers an understanding of feeling as a measure of one's limits and partial perspective. In this way, contemplative pedagogy unlocks situated knowledge's dual structure of situated knowing and what I call "situated feeling." I explore recent discussions of emotion in the field, such as Micciche's "rhetorics of emotion," and argue for situated feeling instead of these performative alternatives, which too often establish the body as an empty stage, not a material agent. Following yoga, I argue for a contemplative understanding of feeling as both *in* bodies and as relational and connective. Viewing emotion from a contemplative perspective frees us to teach emotional awareness as part of the writing process so that writers learn receptivity to their own and others' situated feelings. Far from promoting solipsism, attending to situated feeling attunes us to others and to the outside world of matter as it underscores the physicality of our knowing processes and the idea that understanding is itself material, not simply cerebral, in nature.

The third and final interchapter argues that writers can learn emotional flexibility through the yoga practice of breath control, or *pranayama,* which is understood to be a means of accessing and monitoring emotion. I analyze students' writing products and their reflective statements about their writing processes to show how *pranayama* can not only enrich their felt experience of the writing process and the physical ease and comfort with which they write but can also attune them to the materiality of knowledge making and the ways their emotions are implicated in this process. Students who use *pranayama* as a regular composing ritual begin to appreciate the body as a site of learning and begin to approach writing as a somatic experience. And students who self-consciously engage in these embodied writing practices develop, in turn, a greater metacognitive awareness of the writing process, reflected in their writings about writing. As students breathe their way into writing, they place new value on observing the writing process as it unfolds, documenting and analyzing the felt experience of composing, which helps them become more generative and reflective writers. Particularly, students' increased mindfulness and flexibility results in developed focus and advanced coping mechanisms to deal with the negative emotions of the writing process. To illustrate how writers can increase their resilience and emotional flexibility by practicing yoga, I examine students' writings for the ways they connect breath and emotion and draw on studies of yoga to support their connections.

Finally, my Conclusion returns to the opening narrative of the prologue, creating less a tidy resolution and more a reminder of the circularity we must embrace as contemplative practitioners of writing and yoga. Reflecting on the practice of chanting at the end of yoga sessions, which I have completed many times as both a student of yoga and a teacher of writing, reminds me to leave my manuscript as I leave my practice of yoga: by acknowledging the ending as a beginning and as a point of union between bodies who have come together and leave each other with respect and compassion. It is on this note of connection and promise that I end.

CHAPTER ONE: THE WRITING YOGI: LESSONS FOR EMBODIED CHANGE

> [It's] not that I always write about the body, though I often do, but that I always write, consciously, as a body. (This quality more than any other, I think, exiles my work from conventional academic discourse. The guys may be writing with the pen/penis, but they pretend to keep it in their pants.
> —Nancy Mairs, *Waist-High in the World*

Mairs is helpful when thinking about what it means to write "as a body." In the quote from my epigraph, Mairs acknowledges three major consequences of self-consciously negotiating the writing process as a material endeavor: first, when we acknowledge that writing always springs from our material placement, we add authority and transparency to our compositions, no matter how explicitly our content references our body; second, in this process, we necessarily move beyond the rules and structures of "conventional academic discourse;" and third, this movement engages us in a feminist endeavor that disturbs the ways patriarchal power is enforced by a malestream tendency to erase the writer's materiality in order to create an illusion of objectivity. To write as a body in the ways Mairs describes means disrupting the objectification and marginalization—in other words feminization—of bodies in the academe. No longer is distance from the body a prerequisite to truth; instead, proximity lends persuasiveness.

To understand embodiment as a central facet of feminist composition pedagogy, we must follow the lead of writers like Mairs and accept our bodies as flesh and text. In this chapter, I argue that contemplative writing pedagogy is the best means of achieving this goal while remaining mindful of the consequences of attending to writing bodies. Mairs is an example of a writer who has a greater than usual awareness of her writing body. The quote I use to open this chapter is from her Waist-High in the World, which in title and content fronts this author's literal perspective on the world, her embodied and partial "perpetual view, from the height of an erect adult's waist" (1996, p. 16). Mairs enacts a method of embodied writing in her text such that situatedness and perspective are always understood as material and connected to her writing body; notably, they are not simply convenient metaphors for theorizing.

Mairs' perspective is literally one from the margins because her voice resounds from the seat of her wheelchair. She explains the consequences of this "waist-high" positioning:

> "[m]arginality" thus means something altogether different to me from what it means to the social theorists. It is no metaphor for the power relations between one group of human beings and another but a literal description of where I stand (figuratively speaking): over here, on the edge, out of bounds, beneath your notice. I embody the metaphors (1996, p. 59)

Sitting waist-high in the world isn't a prerequisite for embodied writing, but it does make Mairs mindfully aware of how writing comes just as much from the placement of her fleshy body—sometimes in a wheelchair, sometimes placed on the toilet by her husband—as her cultural and historical orientation. Ours does too, although we can "stand" to ignore this fact because of our able-bodiness.

Because bodies and language unfold to reveal each other, Mairs' material reality influences her semiotic understandings and choices. Mairs' recognition of her embodied subjectivity changes how she chooses to reconstruct her world discursively as she finds less value in normative constructions. Mairs states a preference for calling herself a "cripple" against the wishes of rhetorically-sensitive, politically-correct individuals who understand the power of language to construct the world. She argues that their reconstruction of her world through such "PC" terms as individuals with "differing abilities" do not represent her embodied reality:

> "Mobility impaired," the euphemizers would call me, as through a surfeit of syllables could soften my reality. No such luck. I still can't sit up in bed, can't take an unaided step, can't dress myself, can't open doors (and I get damned sick of waiting in the loo until some other woman needs to pee and opens the door for me). (1996, p. 13)

To deny Mairs' physical reality is to deny her selfhood and her writing body. Pointing out the social construction of disability does little to change her reality of sitting impatiently in the bathroom hoping for someone to open the door.

Mairs serves as a powerful reminder that while mapping out bodies rhetorically may help us to recognize our cultural construction and the shaping power of language, we cannot lose sight of our very real corporeality. Within the field of composition studies, there are few pedagogical approaches we can easily follow to reintroduce the tension of the living, organic body as Mairs does within disability studies—and even fewer that respect the kind of embodied self-reflexivity Mairs demonstrates. We can, however, find ways to bring the productive tension of the writing body to bear on composition praxis by approaching this body through the lens of contemplative pedagogy and practices like yoga. Disability studies and contemplative pedagogy may seem strange bedfellows at first glance, but they share a common focus on respecting the body where and as it is. And, just as disability studies was strengthened by overt attention to disability's intersections with gender (a premise upon which Rosemarie Garland-Thomson's work revolves: see, for instance, Extraordinary Bodies (1996)), so too can contemplative pedagogies be made stronger for their explicit uptake of feminisms.

Contemplative pedagogies stress embodied self-reflexivity, or the ways the body is an anchor of our self-awareness and can be used as a tool of executing and monitoring this reflexive-reflective attention. The ways contemplative pedagogy forwards an integrative approach to education that addresses students as whole beings, bodies, hearts and minds, leads contemplative educator Zajonc to assert that contemplative educators are "engaged in a revolutionary enterprise" that has the power to radically transform higher education (2010, p. 91). The body is the lynchpin for connection: because the embodied self is partial, she can join others without claiming to be them or erasing their difference. While we tend to approach disability/ race/class/gender as embodied barriers within Western rhetorical pedagogies, contemplative pedagogies see these as bridges to connection. Even when coupled with a heightened awareness of the social dimensions of learning and knowing, what contemplative pedagogies they yet need is a deepened awareness of the feminist nature of such attention. As of yet, contemplative pedagogies are often unaware of the ways reclaiming the body in our classrooms is an overtly feminist act since women typically have been objectified as bodies and emptied as minds in Western culture and education. Consequently, my efforts in this chapter will be aimed at developing a theoretical grounding for a feminist-minded contemplative writing pedagogy that constructs the writer as an embodied imaginer in the ways I outline in my introduction and to the ends of respecting the writing body Mairs pinpoints.

Finding sustainable ways to understand this body, or what remains outside the text, is work that remains to be done on both a theoretical and practical level, according to Sanchez in his recent article on empiricism and identity (2012, p. 236). Sanchez offers a reading of the contemporary moment within composition studies as one that "need[s] more, and different, theory" because "composition's modernist and postmodernist legacies together do not offer enough equipment with which to theorize, examine, and teach writing in contemporary contexts," contexts that have us re-examining the role of the writer's "commonsense materiality" (2012, pp. 235-236). I respond to Sanchez' call for "different theory" by following Haraway to explore what feminist science studies may offer contemplative writing pedagogy in the way of new, feminist-contemplative models of subjectivity to help compositionists move from theories of writing subjects to "writing yogis," a necessary first step in addressing the embodied imagination and approaching the writer and her body with mindfulness in the composition classroom. But first, I explain why such a theoretical move is necessary.

MINDLESS BEHAVIOR

Key to understanding the philosophy of yoga is recognizing its premise that when we cultivate mindfulness of our thoughts and feelings, we can choose our behaviors and move beyond the habitual action-reaction cycle, which dictates how we tend to respond to situations. A re-theorization of the writing subject as a writing yogi, a contemplative writer skilled in embodied imagining, is needed in composition studies precisely because the dominant action-reaction chain that dictates how we approach students' and teachers' subjectivity is unresponsive to matter, and mindlessly so. My attempts in this chapter to re-theorize the writer as a writing yogi can be seen as applications of mindfulness from the inside, then, as they pause, listen and respond judiciously in order to create a transformation of self through awareness.

Our mindless or taken-for-granted reaction to matter currently tends to follow the logic James Berlin set forward in his theories of social constructivist pedagogy, reactions themselves to poststructuralist theory. While no longer representative of the cutting edge work in our field, any inquiry into the presence of writing bodies must account for social constructivist pedagogies if only because of the boundaries they have set for what might come next, of what we can build from critical theory. In these theories, Berlin misses the ways the body secures our epistemological perspective with sweeping statements regarding the totality of social construction. Because others have persuasively criticized Berlin's theories on these grounds (see Fleckenstein's Writing Bodies, in particular), I will limit my comments here. Defending the logic of social epistemicism, Berlin asserts that "the symbolic includes the empirical because all reality, all knowledge, is a linguistic construct" (1987, p. 166). While no idealist, Berlin may not outright deny the existence of matter, but he seems to find enough reason to dismiss any agentive status or genuine role in construction it may have. If nature, and the body in turn, can never be known in itself because culture is always mediating it, then for Berlin nature is just another word for culture, and real agency lies in constructivist narratives:

> [T]he distinction between nature and culture can never be determined with certainty. The interventions of culture prevent humans from ever knowing nature-in-itself. In other words, experiences of the material are always mediated by signifying practices. Only through language do we know and act upon the conditions of our experience—conditions that are socially constructed, again through the agency of discourse. (2003, p. 76)

Taken together, Berlin's dismissal of matter for discourse reframes situatedness as an intellectual negotiation referring to cultural and historical placement. Rather than seeing the lack of certain boundaries between the natural and the cultural as liberating and as a way to complicate subjectivity via materiality, as the contemplative does, he places meaning and value in discursive constitution. In other words, Berlin, a master policer of boundaries, seems to want closure whereas mindfulness dictates openness. The body and flesh of the writer are dually edged out. Our commonplaces have encouraged a willful ignorance of matter and our pedagogies have, in turn, left the materiality of teachers and students to the domain outside the classroom.

Discourse-community constructivists like David Bartholomae have also overlooked the body's role in situatedness with arguments about how student writers must (and can) so displace themselves from their material circumstances and enfleshed existence in order to appropriate an authoritative academic persona that will allow them the voice needed to be heard in the academy (Inventing the University). As with Berlin, the problem here is not the demystification of academic discourse but the disembodied presumption. These figurations of appropriation are incomplete without a body to literally place the process or flesh to account for it.

Berlin and Bartholomae remain touchstones for anyone interested in tracing the effects of social constructionist theory over the years, but, of course, as a field, we've moved beyond the initial foundation they laid. Yet, interruptions and complications of their early theories have often not moved us much closer to minding matter. Thomas Newkirk's critiques of critical pedagogy's heavy focus on students' transformation address positioning more explicitly but do so mostly on a figurative level. Newkirk finds appropriation models problematic because they ask students to take on not just a discourse but to "impersonate" a whole new situatedness: when

> students in their late teens and early 20s are asked to engage with texts written for much older readers. An eighteen-year-old reading Foucault for the first time must pretend mightily, appearing to possess the background knowledge, interests, and concerns of an older, invariably more sophisticated (or disillusioned) implied reader. (2004, p. 253)

Newkirk's critique is persuasive but incomplete. He helpfully locates appropriation and ties it to the situatedness of the writer, but still he explains situatedness mostly in discursive terms: students "pretend" by faking a mindset, an attitude. When we view Newkirk's critique from a feminist contemplative perspective, we see that in the appropriation model, we are asking students not only to take on a new discourse but also a materiality not their own, pretending themselves into other (imagined) bodies deemed authoritative or dominant, in turn, willing away their own. Newkirk thus similarly dismisses the inexorable connection between thinking and physical being.

Jane Hindman's mixed-form, academic and autobiographical self-portrait in Making Writing Matter shows the deleterious effects of the double appropriation of matter and language when attempting to assert authority within academic writing—in her case, the professional discourse community of composition studies. Reflecting on the limits of academic discourse to represent her situated subjectivity, Hindman argues that she is not just rhetorically constructed as an alcoholic by the master narrative of Alcoholics Anonymous, but that there is a real, bodily way in which she was already an alcoholic before she ever made the choice to discursively construct herself as such (2001, p. 98). To ask her to take on another subjectivity not uniquely embodied in this way is to do great damage to her inner life and her writing identity and their connections to her physical beingness. It is akin to viewing Mairs' marginality in linguistic but not literal terms.

By viewing Hindman's critique through Haraway, we can see how the problematic tendency to will away the organic body through the process of writing is endemic to the entire university, not only our field, and how this tendency is entangled with the epistemic function of academic discourse and guaranteed by its history. Responding to Sandra Harding's The Science Question in Feminism, Haraway argues that the academy's reliance on the scientific method and its partner-in-power, academic discourse, has provided a patriarchal backdrop that has been used to deny the power of materiality by assessing it a limitation, forever abjecting it to the realm of the feminine. If women have been their bodies in Western culture, men, in turn, have been "freed" to adopt a transcendent and hence disembodied subject position that ensures the objectivity of the knowledge they work to produce.

Haraway elsewhere draws on Steven Shapin and Simon Schaffer's Leviathan and the Air Pump: Hobbes, Boyle and the Experimental Life to argue that this division was solidified by seventeenth century narratives of the Scientific Revolution, wherein men constructed themselves via the scientific method as "modest witnesses," or subjects who could enact intellectual modesty by witnessing reality without implicating themselves in it. What marks the traditional modest witness is that he remains unmarked, acting merely as a "ventriloquist for the object world, adding nothing from his mere opinions, from his biasing embodiment. And so he is endowed with the remarkable power to establish facts" (1997, p. 24), according to Haraway. Rather than voicing from an invested, personal stance, he takes on the role of speaking for the object world, denying the need to voice with the world. Matter remains passive, silent, inactive—a resource from which knowledge can be made but never itself agentive in the making. This is the motivation for the will to discursivity that remains a feature of academic knowledge-making procedures, including the forms of academic discourse our writing pedagogies validate today. As we approach Bartholomae and Newkirk through Haraway, we see that our very understanding of how students come to appropriate academic discourse is based on the concomitant silencing of their bodies.

The separation "of expert knowledge from mere opinion as legitimating knowledge for ways of life … [is a] founding gesture of what we call modernity" (Haraway, 1997, p. 24), and it is one that has continued to hold sway up through contemporary times. This is evident through the continued valuation of a disembodied subject position within knowledge production and also in the writing technologies we have inherited. Because the knowledge obtained from the experimental method was disseminated through written reports, a rhetoric of the modest witness was created alongside this new subjectivity, according to Haraway's feminist historical account. This modest rhetoric was conceived of as a "'naked' way of writing,' unadorned, factual, compelling," laying the way for contemporary academic discourse. "Only through such naked writing could the facts shine through, unclouded by the flourishes of any human author" (Haraway, 1997, p. 26). Writing, out of necessity, was seen as a technology that could be evacuated of subjective partiality, able to provide a transparent and neutral recording of the scientist's or academic's ventriloquist voice. Writing thus became and remains a central part of the methodological apparatus for establishing scientific fact, ordering nature through manageable chunks of transcribed knowledge (Haraway, 1997, p. 26). Observational, scientific reports and claim-driven, academic arguments may retain many differences—such as the attempt to foreground the evidential framework for a claim in arguments—but they are united in their preference for the disembodied modest witness as invoked author. Both kinds of writing value the kind of substantiated proof that takes the writer's personal beliefs, self interests and embodied perspectives as factors that can be transcended in the pursuit of knowledge or in the recognition of the social construction of the self.

The transparent tale and the disinterested, modest observer remain features of recognizable scientific and (therefore) mainstream academic discourse to this day. We have inherited the value of "naked writing," or author-evacuated writing. Even in our own rhetorically-sensitive field, the emotive and experiential self, often (mis)understood to be the personal self of expressivism, is feminized, and granted significantly less epistemological agency, if any at all, than the "modest" academic arguer, the "witnessing" critical intellectual, who furnishes appropriately impersonal, substantiated evidence and displays rationality to make his claims (for an interesting analysis of how this preference plays out in our professional writing see Publishing in Rhetoric and Composition (Olson & Taylor, 1997) especially the chapters Person, Position and Style and Gender and Publishing). It is precisely these inherited notions of objectivity in tandem with deep-set Cartesian mind-body dualism that fueled early feminist disruptions of academic discourse by scholars like Tompkins, Olivia Frey and Linda Brodkey.

Tompkin's article, Me and My Shadow actualizes the struggle between the personal, subjective self, who is to be seen not heard, and the professional, disembodied witness, called to the stand for a kind of modest testimony untainted by the body. Tompkins highlights these subject positions:

> There are two voices inside me .... These beings exist separately but not apart. One writes for professional journals, the other in diaries, late at night. One uses words like "context" and "intelligibility," likes to win arguments, see her name in print, and give graduate students hardheaded advice. The other has hardly been heard from. (1987, p. 169)

Like Brodkey in "Writing on the Bias," Tompkins asserts that in reality the split is a false one, a separation that keeps us from recognizing the embodied and embedded personal because of masculinist conventions; or, as Brodkey says, we are blinded from seeing a biased conventional discourse that "feigns objectivity by dressing up its reasons in seemingly unassailable logic and palming off its interest as disinterest—in order to silence arguments from other quarters" (1994, p. 547). Calls to logic usher in the adversarialism Frey targets in her study of professional journals and conferences.

And we may not have advanced as far beyond these early feminist critiques as we'd like to think. More recently, Hindman has argued that our field persistently values the same kind of arhetoricity and objectivity Haraway credits as a holdover from the Scientific Revolution. While we have ostensibly given up on the ideals inherent in "naked writing," or writing that seeks to escape ideology, we have, at the same time, refused the embodiment of the author. In Writing an Important Body of Scholarship (2002) Hindman charges professional academic discourse in composition studies with a phallocentric perpetuation of an epistemology of objectivity, the domain of the traditional modest witness. Academic discourse used and validated by compositionists in their professional writing, which is Hindman's focus, "works to entextualize an abstract body of knowledge and disembody the individual writer" (2002, p. 100), she says, ironically constructing itself as arhetorical. Hindman points out, in short, how positioning ourselves as modest witnesses in our writing confers the "right" kind of authority to our prose, legitimizing the ideas it espouses precisely because it divorces the writer from her material existence, because it allows her to speak for the world rather than with it.

The modest witnessing required here can be productively challenged by the writing yogi's imaginative claim to her body within feminist contemplative pedagogy. Indeed, we can learn a lot about how to approach matter and writing bodies mindfully by looking to the contemplative practice of yoga. Yogis learn three primary lessons through their practice that are useful when re-crafting the writing subject as material and reconnecting the cognitive and physical aspects of the writing process:

1. Our subjectivity is always first embodied. Our bodies are part of our integral selves because our flesh is intelligent and because our mind/consciousness is diffused throughout the body and is not simply located in the brain or head. To recognize ourselves as body-minds is to see our flesh as a source of power and knowledge. It is to become embodied imaginers.
2. The greatest resources we, as body-minds, have in the quest for awareness are practice and experience. Experience advances the initial wanderings of our imagination and therefore begets wisdom and knowledge.
3. Consequently, it is only with and through the body that we can reach a greater awareness of ourselves and, paradoxically, the world around us—matter is the common thread we share with that world and others

in it. Matter is the connective tissue that unifies us with the world so that the yogi's inner turn to the center is simultaneously an unfolding to the external. A journey that accounts for the personal does not, then, dismiss the cultural but refuses to recognize static separations between the two.

To develop mindfulness of matter in these ways entails being open to a shifting web of positioning and relationality wherein we neither ignore postmodernism's focus on linguistic construction and representation, launching us back into early expressivist or Romantic notions of authentic subjectivity, nor do we allow the deterministic contour of strong linguistic constructivism. Aiding the feminist contemplative writer in this journey to reclaim materiality is an understanding of Haraway's feminist subject. This subject sees her body as instrumental in knowledge-making practices, defining herself neither as a "fixed location in a reified body" or as a "body … blank page for social inscriptions" (1991c, pp. 195-197). This embodied subject shows us another way, neither squarely essentialist nor anti-essentialist, one in kindred spirit to the contemplative project.

While Haraway may not intend to write as a contemplative pedagogue, her interest in non-Western spirituality aligns her project with my own. She forwards a mindfulness of matter that allows me to explore an embodied representation of the writer within contemplative writing pedagogy, one that integrates the key understandings of the yogi and practices these with a feminist edge. Mindful yogis practice at their "edge," the challenge place where they can embody new imaginings but do so in ways that are sensitive to their embodied realities at the present moment. In the same way, by pairing Haraway's key points with yoga's, I am practicing pedagogy at the edge and turning mindfulness back on itself, asking contemplative education to be aware of its feminist potential.

By dialoguing contemplative practice with Haraway's theories of epistemology in what remains of this chapter, I will work toward a definition of writing yogis as those writing bodies that are consciously mindful or aware of their materiality, for there are surely bodies that write unaware of or unwilling to accept the terms of their embodiment. The difference is what Mairs targets; the difference produces what I have previously referred to as the embodied imagination. My exploration of writing yogis will hinge on the importance of conscious awareness and will refuse to deny the integrity of particular bodies, who are situated in time and place, but who also feel and experience their embodiment as, in part, an expression of interiority. This is the responsibility of awareness assumed by the writing yogi as embodied imaginer. My efforts in the remainder of this chapter will be extended in the following interchapters with pedagogical discussions of how to live out the theories of writing yogis through contemplative classroom practices. By following Haraway, my hope is to examine the consequences of defining writing and thinking in terms of the absence of the body and to suggest what writing yogis can do to reclaim their writing bodies and embodied imaginations within contemplative pedagogy.

Lesson 1: Replace the Modest Witness with the Writing Yogi—or, Theorizing the Embodied Imaginer

Mairs' creation of an embodied writing subject is based on her tacit knowledge of being a body in the world. By grounding her writing theory in practice, she advances a central value of the contemplative process. For through practice, the yogi is led to a similar, respectful awareness of her materiality that Mairs attains through the experience of her disability. "The physical body … is not something to separate from our mind and soul. We are not supposed to neglect or deny our body as some ascetics suggest. Nor are we to become fixated on our body" states Iyengar in his book, Light on Life (2005, p. 5), where he documents his philosophies of yoga. His point is that we are our bodies, not just that we have them, and that accepting the vulnerability of the body is both a humbling and liberating experience. Iyengar writes within a contemporary tradition of globalized, international yoga that seeks to blend the teachings from ancient yogic texts like the Yoga Sutras with his own understandings as leader of the Iyengar branch of Hatha yoga. His teachings have great merit within the yoga community because they spring from a lifetime of his own experiences of using his own body as an "instrument to know what yoga is" (2005, p. xx). The body teaches if we listen.

Yoga works toward figurative and literal balance and alignment. The point of practicing yoga, including breath awareness, pranayama, meditation, dhyana, and postures, asana, is to help us integrate and align the layers of our embodied being. Only in their alignment will the yogi reach enlightenment and self-realization: "the practice of yoga teaches us to live fully—physically and spiritually—by cultivating each of the various sheaths" toward the end of integration (Iyengar, 2005, p. 5). Asana not only reminds the yogi of her intimate connection to her body but also teaches her to harness the totality of her awareness by learning to work with and through the body: it becomes the source of her self-realization. And so, in learning her body, she learns the nature of the material world: "If you learn a lot of little things, one day you may end up knowing a big thing" (Iyengar, 2005, p. 14).

Iyengar's statements regarding the centrality of the body in creating knowledge and developing awareness detail the first lesson yogis learn through their practice, as outlined at the conclusion of the last section of this chapter: our subjectivity is always first embodied. Not only are our bodies part of our integral selves, but they are also intelligent since the mind is diffused throughout our physical being. If Western traditions tend to see our brain as synonymous with the mind or consciousness, yoga sees the mind as diffused throughout our material being and not simply located in the head. To recognize ourselves in this way as body-minds is to see our flesh as a source of power and knowledge. Because the thinking and being sheaths of our bodies have "no tangible frontiers" (Iyengar, 2005, p. 6), the journey of the writing yogi is to become aware of the intricacies of the body and the importance of claiming it. Because of her interest in Indian spirituality and non-Western rhetorics, Haraway advocates a similar awareness that comes from recognizing the body as an epistemic origin. In theorizing the contemplative body with her, we can bring feminist mindfulness to contemplative writing pedagogy.

Haraway fully recognizes that while women everywhere have specifically been the "embodied others, who are not allowed not to have a body," feminists should neither simply take on the masculinist subject position of the modest witness in order to be heard nor reactively ignore the body (1991c, p. 183). With the objectifying backdrop we have inherited, Haraway argues it is understandable why so many feminists across disciplines have adopted social constructivist thinking, which use the great equalizer of rhetoric to show the historical, contingent nature of truth. With objectivity dismantled, oppressive power structures are revealed and the inherent rhetoricity of the body is questioned. Haraway finds these poststructural narratives of knowledge-making limiting, since they don't provide adequate grounding for a pragmatic account of the real world (1991c, p. 187). Too many grievously ignore the reality of matter and our flesh in order to secure the epistemological superiority of the modest witness.

Haraway provides an alternative to these narratives by dismantling the modest subject's source of power: vision. She intentionally reclaims vision as the central metaphor to frame her feminist epistemology, stealing it away from the masculinist "cannibal-eye" (1991a, p. 180) or phallocentric psychoanalytical significations of lack and recasts it so that "we might become answerable for what we learn how to see" (1991c, p. 190). The confusing syntax in Haraway's formulation subtly reminds us of the simultaneous naturalness of vision and its social character, as we are taught how to see and what to value in our lines of sight (1991c, p. 190). Queering the traditional understanding of vision as disembodied means for her exchanging lofty notions of transcendent vision for grounded ones. Because there is no unmediated sight, no acultural or immaterial means of seeing, the process is never innocent. Haraway points out the obvious—our vision is always connected to a body. This is a body that is not only marked by culture but is part of a material world in which is it locatable, partial and agentive.

Hers is a "feminist writing of the body" in which "[t]he moral is simple: only partial perspective promises objective vision" (1991c, pp. 189-190). Just what kind of objectivity this entails, I will turn to in a moment. Haraway takes pains to insist that what we can see is limited by our body's composition even if, at the same time, the meaning we can make of our worlds is limited by the cultural and ideological apparatuses we have internalized. "What we learn how to see" stresses to readers that it is just as important to accept the corporeal construction of our visual images, and thus the agentive status of our bodies, as it is to acknowledge the cultural conditioning that enables us to makes sense of what our eyes see. As artists know well, the camera constructs as much as it records. But as those who wear glasses or contacts know just as well, sight is contingent on the body's own agency.

Thusly recasting the metaphor of vision, Haraway's mutated modest witness exchanges the self-effacement of previous versions for self-awareness of her partiality and non-innocence. This new modest witness "insists on situatedness, where location is itself a complex construction as well as inheritance ... [t]he modest witness is the only one who can be engaged in situated knowledges" (1991a, pp. 160-161). Her modest witness is not modest because she is able to view the subject world from a transcendent, disembodied position; rather, her mutated witness is modest precisely because she can only appeal to knowledge from a particular personal, embodied location, a certain material placement of being in/with the world, never above it. From a contemplative perspective, Haraway roots the modest witness in the realm of the material, so that knowing is anchored equally in the cognitive and the material and is brought together through the medium of experience. In sum, Haraway's take on feminist vision helps to bring the fleshy knower into view and testifies to her role in the construction of what is (and can be) seen. It further affirms the responsibilities inherent in understanding the process of seeing as associative, social and relational. Literally and metaphorically, this is a kind of connected seeing.[5] That is, it replaces detachment with engagement, connection and interaction.

As Haraway's quote indicates, the location of the writer-knower must be understood dualistically: both as a "complex construction" as well as an "inheritance." That is, situatedness, the condition of literally being placed somewhere in the world, rests not only on deconstructing and understanding the linguistic web of construction that gives meaning to our historical and cultural placement but also on recognizing our inheritance, our birthright. This includes the material conditions into which we are brought, the real world that supports our organic bodies and the legacy of our flesh. The immediate implication for contemplative pedagogy is the recognition of how the body is instrumental to knowledge, for it is only with and through it that we can come to know or create meaning at all. This is our material heritage as human beings. And while this process affirms the integrity of the individual, it is also a process that connects the individual to other bodies. As we begin to see, the embodied imaginer who engages in local knowledge-making is differentiated by her place in the world as she self-consciously locates herself within it and is inextricably tied to it by awareness of her organic matter, her flesh. Contemplative pedagogy energizes this awareness by understanding it as mindfulness so that the writing yogi does not only maintain focus on her immediate experiences but also faces those experiences openly and with curiosity not hasty judgment.

Replacing transcendence with an embrace of the real does not mean that truth is dismissed in knowledge-making, just redefined. As Haraway states in her autobiographical interview in How Like a Leaf, her "modest witness is about telling the truth—giving reliable testimony—while eschewing the addictive narcotic of transcendental foundations" (Haraway & Goodeve, 2000, p. 158). The loss of transcendence is precisely what figures in Haraway's mutated version of the modest witness as she later goes on to explain:

> I retain the figuration of "modesty" because what will count as modesty now is precisely what is at issue. There is the kind of modesty that makes you disappear and there is the kind that enhances your credibility. Female modesty has been about being out of the way while masculine modesty has been about being a credible witness. And then there is the kind of feminist modesty that I am arguing for here (not feminine), which is about a kind of immersion in the world of technoscience where you ask a hard intersection of questions about race, class, gender, sex with the goal of making a difference in the real, "material-semiotic" world. (Haraway & Goodeve, 2000, p. 159)

Modesty here is defined in opposition to the arrogance of closure and in tandem with understanding one's limits and one's partial perspective. This is a modesty brought on by humility not mastery. Haraway is quick to point out that this kind of sensitivity to situatedness, of partiality of perspective, is powerful because it remains accountable to the material world and to real people. It is this kind of modesty that may help us to redefine our goals of social responsibility within composition to include the conditions of corporeality.

When Haraway's concept is placed within the framework of feminist contemplative writing pedagogy, I suggest that the feminist modest witness becomes the writing yogi who utilizes the skill of embodied imagining. As a tool for inquiry, the embodied imagination is an introspective skill that directs the writer's awareness to the ways knowledge of the external world is linked to self-knowledge. It also insists that mindfulness of bodily sensations and feelings can increase our reflective and reflexive capacities. Iyengar states that yogis are transformed in their contemplative practice of asana and pranayama which "does not just change the ways we see things; it transforms the person who sees" (2005, p. xxi). In turn, the writing yogi who self-consciously claims her embodiment is transformed by a mindfulness of matter that begins with her own body and extends toward other bodies in the world. I outline the consequences of this process for the first-year writing student in the following interchapter. Here, I stress that the writing yogi begins to respect and to take into account how the construction of present realities and future possibilities is based on the knowledge she constructs from experience as well as her affective positions toward other bodies as a result of these experiences. The writing yogi respects her practice as one that creates "knowledge and elevates it to wisdom" by exercising her embodied imagination (Iyengar, 2005, p. xxi). She recognizes intimately that imaginings always occur in the context of material environments and within the frame of her flesh. Our bodies must embrace and enact the dreams and ideas of our intellect for them to mean and to be acted upon.

Through her integrated practice of yoga and writing, the writing yogi recognizes that different bodies produce varying bodies of knowledge and that the expression of a pose or idea may look quite different from one mat to the next, from one paper to the next. Rather than separating, these differences join the embodied imaginer in a humility "that enhances [her] credibility" (Haraway & Goodeve, 2000, p. 159) to others and to nature since, like any one fleshy body, any one body of knowledge is essentially unfinished. Importantly, like Haraway's mutated modest witness, the writing yogi is modest because she recognizes her intimate connection with the world of matter and the relationship between spirit and nature in which neither are rejected even as they are seen "inseparably joined like earth and sky are joined on the horizon" (Iyengar, 2005, p. xxiii). If in Haraway's version of feminist modesty we reclaim the body and refuse transcendence, in kindred spirit, the "modest" writing yogi remains connected yet refuses to lose her center like any other experienced yogi: "In a perfect asana, performed meditatively and with a sustained current of concentration, the self assumes its perfect form, its integrity being beyond reproach" (Iyengar, 2005, p. 14).

The stress I place on the integrity of the self, based on Haraway's theories and the tradition of yoga, differentiates my concept of the writing yogi from the somatic mind as it has been theorized previously in our field. In "Writing Bodies: Somatic Mind in Composition Studies," Fleckenstein asks compositionists to work toward embodied discourse by accepting the concept of the somatic mind, which is to view the mind and body as resolved into a single entity with permeable boundaries. Fleckenstein draws from cultural anthropologist Gregory Bateson to define the somatic mind as "tangible location plus being. It is being-in-a-material place. Both organism and place can only be identified by their immanence within each other" (1999, p. 286). I am arguing for a similarly embodied and connective, but not identical, concept here.

Fleckenstein attempts to get at the writing body through the somatic mind, so that the experience of embodiment she targets is embodiment as placement in external place and time. As she states, "[s]urvival—ecological, psychological, and political—does not depend on the fate of a discrete, atomistic reproducing organism (or subjectivity) because such an organism does not exist. Instead, what exists (and what survives or expires) is the locatedness of somatic mind" (1999, p. 286). Rather than placing the writer in her body, Fleckenstein defines the writer in the contact between her being and her environment, a kind of spaceless space in the union of these permeable substances. Because Fleckenstein's concept is complex, an example here is helpful. Like I did earlier, Fleckenstein uses Mairs to exemplify her concept:

> From the perspective of a somatic mind, the delimitation of Mairs' being-in-a-material-place includes the person, the wheelchair, and the doorway she struggles to enter. Corporeal certainty is not the human being in the wheelchair (the illusory "I"), but the body, the chair, and the doorway simultaneously. (1999, p. 288)

Corporeal certainty is really uncertainty.

Conceived of ambiguously, Fleckenstein's somatic mind remains problematic for contemplative writing pedagogies. A more contemplative perspective would see Mairs as possessing an experience of corporeality that is as much internal as external. If we see Mairs as a somatic mind, we risk denying her the integrity of individual embodiment, and we lose the complexity of the double gesture I take following both Haraway and contemplative practice. Hypothetically, based on the ways Fleckenstein equalizes Mairs with her environment, we could imagine another woman in a wheelchair positioned in the same doorway at the same moment having the same frustrating experience of inaccessibility. There is a move toward corporeal interchangability and dissipation into surroundings here—a move Mairs herself would discredit, I think. Although Fleckenstein's concept is certainly more complicated than such a simple scenario implies, the fact remains that once we remove the subjectivity of the "I," what Fleckenstein calls "illusory," we lose the integrity of the individual body. And whether or not we lose it to the swirling postmodern mass of discourse or to a vortex of intertextual materialities, we lose the unique experience of what it means to be humanly embodied. What it means to be integral or whole is not to be of one inviolable piece so much as it means, in both Iyengar's and Haraway's paradigm, to be undiminished by our interconnectedness with other subjects and objects. Being differentially-positioned in the world means that as bodies we are in a constant flux with our material environments and with other bodies (a kind of dynamic, material-semiotic situatedness I will turn to in the next section), which is not the same as losing the subjectivity of the embodied "I."

Because we experience materiality as a complex relationship between exteriority and interiority, we cannot simply glide over the fact that being positioned by a doorway, even incorporating that too-small doorway into our sense of self at the moment of struggle is different than losing our autonomy or corporeal certainty to the doorway or merging our agency with it. As Haraway states, our embodiment is not simply fixed "in a reified body" but neither is it a "blank page" for other inscriptions, be they material or social (1991c, pp. 195-197). So while I agree that our body boundaries are permeable and our experiences of embodiment include our material environments and are most certainly shaped by our situatedness, I wish to keep a space for body integrity and interiority in my understanding of contemplative writing yogis. For me, this is a more responsible conception since the door cannot experience Mairs as she can it.

Marilyn M. Cooper addresses this problem of agency in her recent Rhetorical Agency as Emergent and Enacted when she argues, "[w]e experience ourselves as causal agents, and any theory of agency needs somehow to account for that experience. And we need to hold ourselves and others responsible for what we do" (2011, p. 437). In this article, Cooper argues for an interactional model of causation, one that accounts for the ways

> an orator does not coerce; he merely puts words into the air. In the brief moments of conscious or unconscious reflection that occur while we listen to a sales pitch or a campaign speech, an active process of evaluation and assimilation occurs in our minds …. When someone sits back and decides, "All right, you have persuaded me," he is not merely describing

> something that has happened to him. In spite of the grammar, he is describing something he has done. (2011, p. 437)

What this scene gets at is Cooper's desire to construe agency as "emergent" (2011 p. 421), as a product of relations and actions, whether conscious or unconscious, and not of simple causation wherein a certain action causes a particular effect in linear fashion. Cooper's understanding of agency as emergent is congruent with a contemplative emphasis on the agency of movement; however, her assumption that if agency is emergent and mobile, it can never rest in an individual is not harmonious—for the same reasons the somatic mind is not—with the contemplative approach I present here.

For in this contemplative approach, the objects and subjects of positioning are not reducible to each other, but are rather always embracing each other as the yogi simultaneously embraces her center and her environment. In his postmodern study of yoga and Buddhist philosophy, George Kalamaras notes that

> [p]aradoxically, the yogi, through various meditative practices, withdraws consciousness from the periphery of the body in ways which heighten the inner sensorium; in total intimacy with a "center" of awareness, then, the advanced mediator's consciousness expands to embrace the immensity of the universe, moving beyond all awareness of limitation, psychological borders, or psychic "circumference." (1997, p. 9)

This never diminishes the integrality of the individual or her ability to consciously act in the world—even if she recognizes her ability to produce effects on that world is as much imaginative as it is real. I will take this argument up once more in my third chapter when I discuss how the acts of extension and expansion allow us to understand embodiment as both an experience of interiority as well as exteriority. In this chapter, I will revisit the concept of integrity once more in the final section by attending to Harway's notion of companion species. But first, I explore the connections between the embodied imagination and Haraway's concept of situatedness.

Lesson 2: Writing Yogis Embrace Situated Knowledge

So what then defines the partial, modest knowledge of the feminist witness or embodied imaginer? Situated knowledge, a paradoxical "embodied objectivity" (1991c, p. 188) is defined as what will allow for a feminist retooling of the knowledge-making process while not discounting the reality of the real or the materiality of the author-actor. This term is meant to underscore just how central our embodied experience is; how knowledge, like the body, is always locatable and always partial. Indeed, situated knowledge rests on the subject's fleshiness, on her inherent embodiment as part of the organic world. Embodiment in this formulation takes on the meaning of dynamically embedded not statically bound. Haraway defines situated knowledges as "marked knowledges" (1991b, p. 111) meaning that they are projects of knowing from the "somewhere" of the embodied subject as opposed to the "nowhere" of traditional empiricism or the "everywhere" of postmodernism (1991c, pp. 188-191). Emphasizing the somatic prerequisite of knowing Haraway states,

> We need to learn in our bodies, endowed with primate colour and stereoscopic vision, how to attach the objective to our theoretical and political scanners in order to name where we are and are not, in dimensions of mental and physical space we hardly know how to name. So, not perversely, objectivity turns out to be about particular and specific embodiment, and definitely not about the false vision promising transcendence of all limits and responsibility .... This is an objective vision that initiates, rather than closes off. (1991c, p. 190)

To learn in and with our bodies means we must first accept that they are integral to the way we produce and understand meaning. The Achilles heel of so many other theories of knowledge production is precisely their assumption that we can rise above our material beingness. Naming "where we are not" entails exactly the opposite.

Haraway's call to learn in our bodies is realized by contemplative pedagogies that advance learned mindfulness through the practice of yoga. "Yoga is something you do" Iyengar tells us, "a conceptual understanding of what we are trying to do is vital, as long as we do not imagine that it is a substitute for practice" (2005, p. 108). Yoga teaches us to recognize and reflexively inhabit our embodiment "to name where we are [and are] not," just as Haraway invites us to do. Like Haraway, Iyengar encourages us to imagine our goals and the future outcomes of our practice, but he warns us to not take such imaginings as reality until they are also embodied. We embody through practice just as we create knowledge through experience. Situated knowledge is exactly what yogis create on their mats when they practice asana and pranayama, learning their "particular and specific embodiment" and therein understanding how their bodies influence the knowledge they make. Because they recognize this, yogis often speak of the problems created when comparing or judging one's version of a particular pose with another's. Each body is different, located in time and space uniquely, which manifests an integral interiority and exteriority that cannot be reduced to another's. Thus, my virkasana, or tree pose, will look different than another yogi's; to expect sameness is to deny our particular embodiments and might lead to injury. Learning yoga therefore becomes a way for writers to begin to value situated, and not transcendent, knowledge: "in this way, the practice of asana, performed with the involvement of all elements of our being, awakens and sharpens intelligence until it is integrated with our senses …. All of our bones, flesh, joints, fibers, ligaments, senses, mind and intelligence are harnessed" (Iyengar, 2005, p. 14). Engaging our flesh leads to deeper, more impactful learning and respect for locatedness.

Objectivity (redefined as local and revisable) is still a factor here; there is truth, however situated, to be told. Our naming processes—including the delineation between the subjective and the objective, the personal and the impersonal—have gotten us into trouble and encouraged us to ignore the source when faced with the subject of vision. Meaning rests on specific, embodied features of our selves, such as the literal way we see because of our corporeal makeup (two eyes in the front of our faces, the intake and interpretation of light by our rods and cones) and the meaning we invest in the patterns of diffracted light our eyes can register, as the long quote above from Haraway underscores. But when we recognize our embodiment as essential to meaning making, we begin to realize that vision from nowhere or from everywhere, are equally impossible. Within Haraway's formulations, objectivity is still possible provided that we understand it to be a responsible process of local knowledge-making that always originates from a body located in a material world, not as that which results in the divorce of matter from intellect or the infinite deferments of empty signs. As in yoga, "[t]he self is both perceiver and doer. When I use the word "self" with a small s, I mean the totality of our awareness of who and what we are in a natural state of consciousness" (Iyengar, 2005, p. 14).

Unlike other knowledge processes, which produce independent or "true-in-themselves" facts, situated knowledge "initiates" according to Haraway's same passage above. I understand this to mean that situated knowledge is polyvocal so that it encourages conversations and joint revisions, making it a relational process. It begins a conversation rather than ending it. Recognizing our specific embodiment and, in turn, our partiality encourages us to join with others in order to test our view against others' and to create relational, contextual knowledge. Thus, this conversation extends beyond dialogism as it invites in multiple voices. These factors all add up to what makes Haraway-ian situated knowledge contemplative: because it originates from our body, it is not simply another way of expressing the groundless "contingent" knowledge of other theories. Rather, situated knowledge complicates contingency by embracing history and critically accepting ideology while resolutely maintaining a material connection to fleshy bodies in a real world of matter. These bodies produce similarly embodied truths that connect individuals in webs making them accountable to one another in the flesh.

Lesson 3: Writing Yogis See the World in Terms of Connections

In this way, through situated knowledges we can create "an earth-wide network of connections, including the ability partially to translate knowledges among very different—and power differentiated—communities" (Haraway, 1991c, p. 187).[6] Our embodiment can consequently become something of a common ground, even if we all experience it differently. Without a doubt, the meetings and negotiations with different others are what gives this knowledge its power. The web-like structure of situated knowledge is actually more powerful than the hierarchical structure of the past: "[l]ocal does not mean small or unable to travel" (1991c, p. 161) Haraway reminds us. As a critical and reflexive practice, situated knowledge thereby enacts feminist connected knowing.

Connected knowing values the historical and experiential by taking on a relational orientation to what is being studied by those who are doing the studying—meetings matter. Such knowing procedures are characterized by an acceptance of openness and by a recognition of the need to join with others. In contrast to separate knowers who experience the self as autonomous, connected knowers experience the self as always in relation with others (Belenky, et al., 1973, pp. 113-123). The physical and metaphorical figure of the web is telling of the kind of power situated knowledge and the processes of connected knowing entail. Webs stress the connection of bodies and the inter-relatedness of knowledge; they enable that which is small to have a widespread impact as the ripples of a single tug can be felt throughout the entire structure. They also represent how separate bodies can sometimes feel entrapped by communal representation, highlighting the need for individual nodes. Even if notions of the web allow for responsiveness that hierarchies do not, there are risks in this system of power just like any other. And yet in the web, "[e]ach person—no matter how small—has some potential for power" precisely because of the heightened accountability of being "subject to the actions of others" and others being subject to one's own actions (Belenky et al., 1973, p. 178). This is quite unlike a hierarchical pyramid where one must "move a mountain" to effect substantial change (Belenky et al.,

1973, p. 179). Iyengar describes connected knowing similarly in the language of yoga: "In asana our consciousness spreads throughout the body, eventually diffusing in every cell, creating a complete awareness. Asana is the "broad gateway" that teaches us to discover awareness through our bodies and to keep our bodies "in harmony with nature" (2005 p. 11). It is this focus on connection that characterizes the contemplative.

Contemplative pedagogy theorized through Haraway recognizes that difference itself is not the end; rather, difference implies a partiality that necessitates the joining of the subject with others in order to form coalitions based on affinity not identity.[7] Difference works not just to divide but also to unite. "Some differences are playful; some are poles of world historical systems of domination. 'Epistemology' is about knowing the difference" (1991c, p. 161). Contemplative pedagogy is about working with difference toward a state of balance, starting with the writer's connection between her body and the body of the other.

The yogi understands her body as intimately connected with and as part of a larger world of matter, of nature. Thus, in exploring her "own body, [she is] in fact exploring ... nature itself" (Iyengar, 2005, p. 22). In the tradition of yoga, we, as individual material bodies are a part of nature; nature, or prakrti, is "all that is practical, material, tangible, and incarnate" (Iyengar, 2005, p. 6). Therefore, as I noted earlier, it is only with and through the body that yogis can reach a greater awareness of ourselves and, paradoxically, the world around us, since matter is the common thread we share with that world and others in it. The yogi's inner turn to the center is simultaneously an unfolding to the external. A journey that accounts for the personal does not, then, dismiss the cultural but refuses to recognize separations between the two. "Individual growth is a must, and yoga develops each individual" says Iyengar, "[b]ut your body is an image of the world around you: it is a big international club" (2002, p. 11). Yoga's understanding of the self as prakrti means that not only are we situated in and among the matter of the earth, but that our understanding of the world is always fixed to our placement in it. This doesn't mean that our understanding or placement is static—quite the contrary. The situatedness of our understanding means that like nature, we too are constantly changing. I'd like to put these contemplative understandings in dialogue with Haraway once more to complete the feminist epistemology I'm building in this chapter for contemplative writing pedagogy.

Haraway, like Iyengar, argues that when we talk about bodies, we talk about the world; "our" flesh is the matter of the world. She calls this "significant otherness" and discusses how it changes our relationship to other species, what we might now perceive as companion species. Haraway says, "I go to companion species, although it has been over-coded as cats and dogs .... I think of the

'Cyborg Manifesto' and Companion Species Manifesto as bookends around an interrogation of relationalities where species are in question and where posthuman is misleading" (Haraway & Goodeve, 2000, p. 140). Extending her conversation about the interconnectedness of nature and culture and, therefore, of subjects and objects, The Companion Species Manifesto argues for a mode of kinship that joins together the rights and responsibilities of species. Taking as paradigmatic the relations between dogs and humans, she reconceptualizes human evolution from this ecologically-minded trope of "significant-otherness." Conventionally, we deem those closest to us, our significant others. Suggesting close-bonds between animals and humans, this term enables Haraway to forward a basic argument against anthropocentrism based on a grid of materialism on which humans can be mapped but not independently. Her argument thus extends to include the relational responsibilities of cross-species development and communication. By arguing for humans' and dogs' significant otherness Haraway gives us a language to speak back to "[b]iological and cultural determinism [which are] both instances of misplaced concreteness" (2003, p. 6).

Of herself and her dog, Ms. Cayenne Pepper, she says, "We are, constitutively, companion species. We make each other up, in the flesh" (2002, p. 3). These two, human and animal, are "significantly" other to each other because their constitutional makeup depends on their companionate relations. This is a twist on the conventional process of othering which divorces rather than connects. This entails a radical shift inasmuch as each being must now be seen as literally constituted in its relation to others. Of course there are practical reasons for their connected co-constitution including the balance of athleticism and handling both Cayenne and Haraway need in order to compete in the agility competitions they enter together. But Haraway is after something deeper, to which her final phrase attests. Haraway is not merely speaking of identity politics here, of what we align ourselves with and against as a product of our culture and ideological commitments; rather, this is a body identity that encompasses those politics and goes even further. Selfhood is seen here as a fleshy process in which each body is responsive to the other in terms of a materiality that goes beyond even consciousness, all the way to biology.

It is in terms of biology, which Haraway uses to get at nature without reifying it, that she first frames her usage of "companion." Questioning the effects of her and Cayenne's interactions within Notes from a Sportwriter's Daughter from When Species Meet (2008), Haraway details her Australian Shepherd's quick tongue, which has "swabbed the tissues of my tonsils, with all their eager immune system receptors" leaving her to wonder, "Who knows where my chemical receptors carried her messages, or what she took from my cellular system for distinguishing self from other and blinding outside to inside?" (2008, p. 2). Haraway knows that her questions are purely speculative and that they represent queries most do not think about yet alone pose seriously. But, these questions give her a tangible way to get at her argument that we must be accountable to our materiality and the way that it binds us to others—an accountability our current theories do not provide. Such accountability is forecasted in the etymology of her first term:

> Companion comes from the Latin cum panis, "with bread." Messmates at table are companions. Comrades are political companions. A companion in literary contexts is a vade mecum or handbook like the Oxford Companion to wine or English verse; such companions help readers to consume well …. As a verb, companion is "to consort, to keep company," with sexual and generative connotations always ready to erupt. (2008, p. 17)

Haraway thus pins her notion of companion species to both material conditions of living and "being with" as well as language, showing how both rest on co-constitution and interrelatedness or on "an ongoing 'becoming-with'" (2008, p. 16).

If we understand Harway's figuration of companion species as a means of establishing the centrality of relationships within a feminist materialist epistemology, we not only see the coherence between Iyengar's discussion of the connectedness of all matter by virtue of its belonging to the state of prakarti but we can see the ways significant otherness in Haraway's formulations are implicated in contemplative practices' focus on "reciprocal revelation" (Hart, 2008, p. 236). Contemplative educator Tobin Hart defines reciprocal revelation as the "willingness to really meet and, therefore, be changed by the object of inquiry, whether a new ideas or a new person" (Hart, 2008, p. 236). It is this kind of revelation of our infinite mutability in the face of others that prompts Iyengar to marvel at the openness developed by the yogi who recognizes that "we are a little piece of continual change looking at an infinite quantity of continual change" (2005, p. 7). To understand significant otherness or reciprocal revelation, we must be willing to first acknowledge our interdependence with the larger world of matter, which encompasses but never diminishes us, and second, we must recognize how this requires our full presence in the moment of meeting others, a skill developed by contemplative practice.

Haraway shows us how reciprocal revelation rewrites the history between dogs and humans and in so doing, illustrates what revisionist accounts that forward mutual responsibility and respect might do to "produce a female symbolic where the practice of making meanings is in relationship to each other" (Haraway 1995, p. 56). She details the history of the transformation of wolves into dogs, the first domesticated animals. Attracted by the waste dumps of human settlements, wolves moved ever closer to contact. "By their opportunistic moves, those emergent dogs would be behaviorally and ultimately genetically adapted for reduced tolerance distances, less hair-trigger fright … and more confident parallel occupation of areas also occupied by dangerous humans" (Haraway, 2008, p. 29). The interrelation was further defined when humans began controlling these wolf-dogs' means of reproduction and slowly bred out aggressiveness.

But this is not a one-sided story. As much as people had a part in this story, this is one about co-evolution, not about the mastery of domestication. Haraway argues that humans may have capitalized on the many benefits of the would-be-dogs including their skills at herding and hunting but the animals were certainly agentive as well. Testifying to the limits of our notions of consciousness, Haraway's against-the-grain analysis draws on a study of Russian foxes to argue that these "wolves on their way to becoming dogs might have selected themselves for tameness" (2004, p. 305). Not to be overlooked is wolves' opportunism and "choice" to interrelate in this story; humans, after all, provided food and shelter. To ignore these species' entanglements is to refuse to respect meetings between selves and others—whether they are animals and humans, humans and humans, or minds and bodies. And to acknowledge these entanglements, we must attune our ability to be contemplatively present in the world so that we might respond to it and not simply react.

Haraway uses her discussion of companion species to refine her understanding of subjectivity within her feminist epistemology; in doing so, she brings us even closer to a contemplative subject understood through the lens of prakarti. Because the body is part of a material world that extends far beyond our powers of discursive construction, it refuses to be dominated or written entirely by our narratives and is storied by nature itself. The self she defines can be understood as a yogi: "[s]ince yoga means integration, bringing together, it follows that bringing body and mind together, bringing nature and the seer together, is yoga. Beyond that there is nothing—and everything" (Iyengar, 2002, p. 48). How we get students to begin to see themselves in such integrative ways, as writing yogis, is the subject of my first interchapter.

To reflect companionate duality, Haraway calls subjects material-semiotic agents. By highlighting the material and the linguistic in one term and hooking agency on both, Haraway reminds her reader that this is a subjectivity built on a fundamental dynamic in which we humans have a role in constructing the world, certainly, but not the role. This generative limitation can begin to explain why matter exceeds our discursive constructions and respects the agency given to matter in Eastern philosophies like yoga. The contemplative insight here is that rather than limiting our ability to understand, this web-like approach to knowledge is precisely what allows us to seek situated truth and situated knowledges. For, epistemological meaning rests just as much on materiality as it does on language.

Mairs claims as much in Waist-High in the World when she notes that it is impossible and dangerous to represent her mind as superior to and separate from her failing M.S.-stricken body, as if her body were a mere object that could be divorced from her self. Mairs so interweaves her subjectivity with her body that when speculating about who she would be without her chronic disease she answers, "Literally, no body. I am not 'Nancy + MS,' and no simple subtraction can render me whole" (1996, p. 8). While she recognizes that she can chose to write about topics that don't include her health or explicitly refer to her body, Mairs argues that writing without her body is impossible, that her writing identity is entangled with her material reality (1996, pp. 9-10). Mairs is mindful of the ways she is her body largely because she has to be; she simply does not have the luxury of divorcing her subjectivity from her material reality because her material positing affects the literal, not just figurative, position of her perspective. Importantly, embodied subjectivity is to Mairs constructed as much by her brain chemistry as by cultural configurations of her semiotic tags and biological realities as a "depressed MS sufferer" (1996, p. 42). Calling herself a "creature" of her "biochemistry" (1996, p. 42), Mairs see bodies as more than mere objects of knowledge or that which is merely marked by the discursive, thinking subject. By using Mairs as an instructive example, we can begin to investigate how refusing to give up our fleshiness opens up new avenues of rhetorical power and options of making meaning through the union of language and the body. These are the options feminist contemplative writing pedagogy secures.

INTERCHAPTER ONE: USING "BODY BLOGS" TO EMBODY THE WRITER'S IMAGINATION

> I have never heard of the mind-body experience in my life but at this moment I still feel like writing is a brain thing and not a mind-body thing. There are only two things that you need to write: your brain, and a *hand*.
> —Student blog response

The first step in developing what I am calling the embodied imagination is encouraging student writers to think of themselves as writing yogis, writers who self-consciously embrace their materiality and approach their writing bodies and the writing process with mindfulness. In the last chapter, I explored how we might weave together the contemplative philosophies of yoga with materialist feminism to theorize the presence and domain of writing yogis. In this interchapter, I move theory to practice. What I outline in the following pages is one attempt to get students both to contextualize their writing experiences in terms of their bodies and to conceptualize their bodies as agentive points of mediation between a culture that seeks to mark them in particular ways and a personal, material reality awash with experiences and feelings that can be used to speak back to that culture, particularly through the creation of embodied, situated knowledge. Using a composite account from a series of recent first-year writing courses (referred to here in the singular), I detail the ways feminist contemplative writing pedagogies can make the body visible in the writing classroom and examine the practical consequences of such visibility.

In this course, I developed a double focus on our bodies both as the subject of inquiry and as integral to the writing experience itself. Not only did I want students to investigate the corporeality of the writing process, I also wanted them to imagine the ways they made sense of the world as primarily embodied and, thereby, to complicate their notions of experience and personal knowledge. I hoped that my students would begin to see how their material realties and corporeality helped construct notions of how they understood the world and the ways they created meaning in their writing; I wanted them to become attentive to their fleshiness and to adapt their writing process to admit in elements of feminist contemplative pedagogy, which is receptive to the student writer as an embodied whole. That is, I hoped students would begin seeing themselves as flexible writing bodies, as writing yogis.

I believed that investigating embodiment as a field of study as well as a lived condition would recursively strengthen these abstract and concrete endeavors, lending a pragmatic balance between the two. An investigation into the importance of our flesh itself represents a cultural and theoretical shift in writing studies, making our once untouchable, unacknowledgeable bodies the focus of the writing classroom in ways that do not seek primarily to textualize them. Instead, the cultural body and lived body are here fused into one, at once complicating our rhetorical notions of reading and writing as well as our field's understanding of "the personal" in ways I related within my last chapter. Claiming the personal *as* the "particular and specific embodiment" (Haraway, 1991c, p. 190) that makes meaning-making possible frees a space in which to think about the material-semiotic entanglement of the fleshy body and the cultural body which come together under the full rubric of embodiment—without essentializing this term or reifying the writing body.

In order to work toward a positive and integrative hermeneutic of corporeality, my first challenge lay in helping students reconnect to their bodies in the classroom, bodies that they had been programmed by years of education to ignore when doing academic work. The opening quote in my epigraph to this chapter humorously yet seriously highlights this learned ignorance by pointing to the irony of my student Nikki's ability to articulate the importance of mind *and* hand to the writing process and yet fail to connect the two. By the time we get them, our students have learned to disconnect their intellectual pursuits from their personal bodies, unless they are in physical education classes where the body cannot and need not be pretended away. From the hard plastic chairs in which they are to sit passively, to the rules students are accustomed to follow prior to their college classes (and even in some classes at this level), such as waiting to use the restroom until after class or not eating during class, students have been cultured to ignore and control their bodies when attending to the development of their minds. Prior to concluding that writing was solely a mental endeavor, Nikki, the student quoted in my epigraph, shared a response in her blog that was telling of how student bodies are endlessly trained to "behave" in educational settings. She noted:

> Class is one of those things where my mind is awake (for the most part) and my body just wants to do something, finding the only occasional relief when I raise my hand to answer a

> question. My brain is processing the information that is being said in class while my body is like "I want to move around" and normally responds with my foot tapping. Although, by the end of the first class my brain has had enough for the day as my body is excited to finally move.

Here, the primary body expression my student imagines acceptable in the classroom is the docile one of raising her hand. Aside from calling up Foucauldian images of passive bodies, Nikki's controlled language is telling in the ways it submerges the tug-of-war between body and brain at the same time that it describes it. Her reliance on the "although" that begins the final sentence reproduced in her response belies the ease with which she controls her body, underscoring the involuntary nature of her foot tapping. Also worth note in this response are the action verbs—do, raise, move—that she uses to describe her body even when she is ostensibly telling her reader how her body must remain passive when her mind is "processing information."

Because her brain soon wears out from this processing, she capitulates to her "excited" body after just one class. Even though her body belies her, Nikki has been so well trained that she concludes in a later blog her belief that writing is a purely mental endeavor—the quote in my epigraph—even though she seems to recognize some unfulfilled link between the mental body and physical body in both responses. First-year composition instructors can easily support these learned views by conducting classes in ways that encourage students' passive bodies, such as when we don't spend time openly discussing how our bodies are implicated in the writing and learning process, and when we dismiss the constructive role of the lived body and experience, often a knee-jerk reaction to sidestep the labels "expressivist" and "essentialist." Even so, there are pedagogical means by which we can recover these losses without trapping ourselves within uncomplicated views of language or culture. I am particularly interested in the ways contemplative writing pedagogy, particularly when informed by feminist principles and practices like yoga, can be such a means. Here, I detail the ways I proceeded with small steps toward that end goal.

To work against this learned reaction to dismiss the body and to begin investigating and valuing embodiment within the context of my class, I constructed a series of "body blogs" that asked students to consider how their bodies were implicated in their writing and learning processes. Known to my students at the start of their blogs were the ways we would eventually build off early writings with a sequenced yoga practice integrated into our class, a practice meant to actualize their initial findings and speculations and to move them toward non-dualistic notions of the mental body and physical body within the context of the writing process. I explore this integrated practice of yoga and writing in Interchapters Two and Three. The pedagogical reasoning behind these blogs was fairly simple: if ignoring our bodies is learned, then it can be unlearned as my own development as a yogi suggests. Of course, this "unlearning" is a slow and gradual process that students may initially find strange since it flies in the face of their pervious relationship to their bodies as learners.

As my course unfolded, I had numerous concerns about how to go about such a process of "unlearning" in ways students would find productive; I did not want them to feel they were simply riding a hobby horse of their teacher's; I wanted them to find a personal stake in our journey. I was especially worried about students' negative reactions to a body focused-class. As this experimental course of mine was also a first-year writing requirement for my students, the first of a two-semester sequence at my university, they had no prior knowledge of the course prior to being assigned to my section and were simply placed into my classroom to meet general education requirements. Even if students found themselves drawn to our investigations, I was worried that their interest would wane as they began to discuss their classroom activities with peers and friends enrolled in other writing sections structured around topics and exercises they might view as "safer" or less disruptive of their preconceptions of a composition class. Finally, I was concerned that students would resist sharing information about their bodies, information they might view as private or too personal.

Ultimately, this final fear was baseless, as I have found most students eager to discuss and analyze their bodies—something they hardly get to do reflectively in the context of other courses and, often, in the context of their personal lives. In the latter case, students are often too busy *being* a body to think much about what this means, as I've discovered in my conversations with them. As with other invitations to explore the significance of personal experiences, students are often excited to talk about themselves and engage in a discussion that puts their lives in dialogue with our course themes and texts. Nevertheless, I always do put in place safeguards for reluctant students, including making certain blog posts private (shared just to me) and allowing students to discuss bodies other than their own. These individual blogs were supplemented by public posts on our course blog and, of course, collaborative, real-time classroom discussions.

BODY BLOG PART 1

The only way I felt I could address the first two concerns regarding student resistance to our topic was to plunge in from the very beginning of our class so as to make the investigation into our bodies a steady element of the course. I introduced the first body blog in the first week of class and explained its importance by tying it to the thematic content of our first unit, "Narrating Bodies." I planned this unit to introduce embodiment as a legitimate topic of study in the writing classroom. In it, we read works that put in question our ability to narrate our identities outside the framework of our flesh like Shelly Jackson's My Body: A Wunderkammer, Bridget Booher's Body Map of My Life, Judith Ortiz Cofer's The Story of My Body and Alice Walker's Beauty: When the Other Dancer is the Self. This unit allowed me to set the stage for our course-long investigation of embodiment and to give greater weight to my students' individual, course-long blogs; we were simply finding our own ways to document our writing identities, keeping our field of study, writing, in mind and applying the insights of our authors to our own bodies and writing processes.

The first blog asked students to identify their writing selves, to talk about themselves as writers, characterizing their motivations and habits, and asked them to reflect on how they approached writing. Students were to use their answers to begin thinking through how their bodies shaped their writing habits and habitats. Questions I invited my students to consider included: "What kind of environment do you prefer when you write? When do you like to write and in what positions do you put your body? Do you sit up, lie down, eat, play music, watch TV, etc.? What kind of sensory experiences do you have as a writer, and how do you feel as you write? For instance, if you get stressed, do you notice your leg tapping up and down, or do your hands get clammy? How do your body and mind play off of one another as you write? Does your nose seem to pick up all food smells within a mile radius when you write, distracting you? Or do you get so absorbed, you lose the desire to eat?" Because this response was the first step of many toward encouraging my students to think about themselves as writing bodies, I also requested my students venture a few guesses as to *why* they might work in the ways they described and what they thought about our project of investigating the body-mind connection as writers.

As a corollary part to this blog, I asked my students to complete a more general reflection on their writing experiences, both formal and informal. This is a fairly common assignment in our field, but one with which many students, astonishingly, seemed to have little prior experience. Many students commented upon the fact that they had never before been asked to think about themselves as writers. One student summed up the class' collective surprise by saying, "When given the chance to write about myself as a writer, I was taken aback at first. I've never thought about my writing before … [but] just purposefully did it for school." Having used versions of this general reflection for years in my writing classrooms, I was surprised at their collective experience since metacognition is crucial for writing students' improvement since it engages them in setting goals, tracking accomplishments and weaknesses and generally finding a stake in their writing beyond simply earning a passing grade. If nothing else, students' surprise at being asked to reflect on their writing is a reminder that we need to signal why we assign certain kinds of writing; it may be that my students were asked to reflect in previous writing assignments but that the goals and the language of reflection were hidden within the framework of some larger project.

Keeping these aims in mind, this general reflection also asked students what they thought qualified as "good" writing in college, how that might differ from high school expectations, and what their writing goals were for our class. Not only did this standard reflection provide me a sense of my students' previous writing experiences and them a sense of accountability for their learning in my class, but it also gave us a platform for the main part of the assignment. I instructed those students who could not yet answer how their bodies might be implicated in their writing processes to complete this second reflection first, before thinking through part one of the blog. Many students, even those who had made observations about their writing bodies prior to the blog, found this building-block approach helpful as it allowed them a type of "embodied remembering" experience wherein their initial speculations of how they positioned their bodies and the conditions of their preferred material writing environments were triggered, proven and even built upon.

Not surprisingly, the written responses to the first blogs overwhelmingly described writing as an onerous task to be put off for as long as possible. Many described the writing experience as one of procrastination and eventual pain. At this stage, students had a tendency to approach the notion of being a writing body with disbelief. In fact, I noted students' tendency to rely on an adversarial language of battle to describe their attempts of controlling their bodies when writing. The metaphorical usage of battle as a conceptual map for relations between the body and mind itself points to the ways in which the meaning we make is grounded in our material realities as bodies in the world.[8] At the same time, it propels a conceptual dichotomy between the mind and the body, seeing them as warring factions, specifically in that the reasonable mind must dominate the unruly body.

For instance, one student wrote, "My mind knows that I NEED to sit down, focus, and write a paper, but my body is bored (tapping leg) or hungry and they are in constant battle to win me over while writing a paper." Another female student, Jamie, accounts for this "battle" in her blog's figurative language, equating her flesh with the death of her creativity or writing ability: "Writing for me is solely a mind thing. If I start trying to bring in other senses I'm *done for*, because I automatically get absorbed in whatever sense I'm thinking about and then the writing goes out the window, so to speak. I try not to be aware of the rest of my body while I write because I, clearly, get distracted" (emphasis added). Yet another student describes the way his body betrays him when writing: "I will always get antsy when writing school assignments … so assignment papers are a very painful experience. This is why I dread them so much." It seems at this point students are ready to blame the battle wounds that show up in their papers in the form of undeveloped ideas, disorganized structures and wandering sentences on the ways their bodies disrupted the functions of their perfectly capable minds; viewing these as discontinuous allows them to maintain the Cartesian split between their bodies and minds and to construe weakness as an element of the flesh.

Because they did not view their bodies and minds as continuous or as companion composers of meaning, students at this stage had a hard time connecting the details they shared about their composing habits and embodied writing experiences to their understanding of the writing process. As a result, after detailing the ways their bodies move, bounce, channel their mental energy and fidget when they get tired, my students overwhelmingly concluded their responses with statements referencing how their bodies were *not* part of the writing process. For example, the student above, Jamie, who admits she is "done for" if she thinks about her body while writing and claims writing as purely mental expression states in the same blog that when she writes, she "move[s] around a lot. Like now for instance, I am currently rocking my chair back and forth …. Also when I write I like to hear the click of the keys as I type, I need that auditory sense to be able to type or it just feels weird …. Also when I write I start bouncing one of my legs." And, it is immediately after this sentence that details her body's energy that Jamie claims, "Writing for me is solely a mind thing." That listening to the clicking keyboard keys means she finds comfort *and* creativity in the sensory experience of the writing process doesn't occur to my student in this response and neither does the ways she obviously channels the rocking and bouncing energy of her body, as synched with her mind, to achieve the goals of her writing session. This lack of corporeal self-awareness is further confirmed when Jamie admits in her conclusion to this blog that she is "hyper aware of other bodies when I write. One of my pet peeves is when somebody is reading over my shoulder while I write or type." Other bodies are even more accessible to Jamie than her own. Writing herself into a similarly complex position, Nikki conceded that the body blog

> assignment has allowed me to realize the small things my
> body does while I am writing. Something that I do when I

> write is that my right leg bounces up and down as if it were on a spring board, especially when I get particularly into what I am writing or I am somewhat stumped. Also I tend to hit two of my teeth together when I am thinking about how I am going to structure the next sentence. I'm not sure how to describe what I am feeling when I write, possibly because when I do write it is as if the computer is sucking up all of my emotion (which in most cases is what I want). I get inspired by a lot of things, but one thing that makes me write on a consistent basis is my short temper. I get mad … extremely mad very quickly and in order to prevent taking it out on some innocent bystander I let my anger out on a piece of paper …. In all honesty before this blog, I have never heard of the mind-body experience in my life but at this moment I still feel like writing is a brain thing and not a mind-body thing. There are only two things that you need to write: your brain, and a hand.

I use the end of this particularly interesting student response as my epigraph to this interchapter precisely because it sums up the contradictory messages these blogs revealed. Students at this stage had plenty to share about their material writing environments and bodily habits but couldn't go so far as to conceptualize or imagine themselves as writing bodies. While she notes the ways her leg bounces and teeth tap together, for instance, Nikki cannot see writing as more than a "brain thing." In short, she, along with her classmates, still found it difficult to claim their embodiment. I chose to include a full version of the above response to show how this was so, even as many of my students seemed to know something fundamental about the workings of embodied narratives, which start at the level of our feelings and emotions. Above, Nikki articulates this felt understanding when she explains how her emotions are a crucial part of the invention stage of writing so that her body literally brings her to the page.

Nikki's response articulates a popular view of emotion as inspiring us to write, even if she cannot yet see how *emotion* is another movement of her body like her chattering teeth and bouncing leg. Hindman claims emotion as a central motivation or "mover" of embodied writing in her article, Making Writing Matter. Hindman, like my student, states that her emotions often propel her to write, taking as case-in-point her sudden and overwhelming anger at hearing her experiences with alcoholism rhetorically-codified and academically-neutralized by conference presenters in ways that denies her embodied experience of being an alcoholic (2001, p. 103). It is this anger that propels her to write

Making Writing Matter, a reflection on the embodied nature of writers and the prose they produce. What these professional and student examples together point out to me is that when we tap into our visceral reactions, we can expect to open the door to feeling as well as thinking processes. But unlike Hindman, who has the authority to introduce contrastive readings via her professional position and public writing forum, Nikki does not (perhaps *cannot* just yet) view her emotional or visceral response as necessary, healthy or potentially constructive. Even if writing does allow Nikki to channel her anger from a physical expression of violence, she wishes to be devoid of feeling: she wants the computer to "suck" up all her emotion. While we can easily read the writing process she describes here as embodied, Nikki's motivation is to feel *less* like a vulnerable body (a liberating move against the tide for Hindman) and *more* like an empty channel, highlighting her wish to control her body as opposed to tapping into it and any accompanying feelings in order to cultivate patient awareness. The comparison between my student and Hindman highlights how, when we view the body as separable from the mind, we take up the cultural baggage that casts the flesh as that which makes us vulnerable instead of that which enables positive action.[9] Contemplative pedagogies, of course, do the opposite: they "addres[s] the whole human being … [reaching] far beyond the conventional goods of learning such as an informed citizenry or an intelligent workforce" (Zajonc, 2010, p. 90).

BODY BLOGS PART TWO AND THREE

If the first blogs were to gauge my students' initial reactions to our investigation of their bodies as central to writing and meaning-making processes, the second and third installments of the body blog were geared toward my attempt to help students work toward an understanding of embodiment in line with those found in Hindman and extended by the feminist writings of Haraway and popular yogic texts like Iyengar's *Light on Life* and *Light on Yoga* (1965), approachable modern tomes of ancient philosophies updated for modern audiences. Embodiment seen from Haraway's feminist lens, as earlier stated, is neither about a "fixed location in a reified body" nor about "the body as anything but a blank page for social inscriptions" (Haraway, 1991, pp. 95-197); rather, it is about the relationality and co-constitutionality of the fleshy, material body, a presence whose situated reality cannot be exhausted by discourse, and the semiotic body, situated and located by means of our discursive mapping practices. Because these mapping practices are constantly changing and our bodies are in constant flux as with the rest of the material world, embodiment is never static and cannot be essentialized within this feminist-contemplative picture.

Showing the kindred nature of feminist theorizing and yogic philosophies, Iyengar, founder of the yoga method that shares his name, says much the same in his own writing about the dynamism between the individual body and the world. Iyengar states that the lived body cannot be conceived of as separate from the material world, both of which are "constantly changing so that we are always looking at nature from a different viewpoint" (2005, p. 7), as our bodies and environments constantly shift, change and adapt. The body I want my students to claim in and through their blogs, following such ideas, is the lived body, which is understood through material dynamism as connecting us to the larger material world of which we remain, through our flesh, an inextricable part. Embodiment is both a social mapping process, signifying and marking our social interactions, *as well as* a material reality. As a result, experience is a way of naming our embodiment, which can never be fully exhausted by discourse since our bodies retain agency both within and beyond our discursive conventions. These body blogs put these ideas in action as they ask students to think about the ways they experienced their bodies as writers and felt the consequences of both their interiority and exteriority unfolding into and onto each other as so many layers of phyllo dough.

To tap into my students' existing knowledge of the reality of their lived bodies, I asked them in the second installment of the body blogs to answer the question, "Beyond writing, how do you otherwise express yourself as a body?" I wanted them to think through the daily movements of their bodies and the kinesthetic knowledge their bodies held when viewed through the lens of the activities in which they actively participated. Central to my whole project was getting students to view body expressiveness as tied to critical writing. I explained to students that "activities" within this context could certainly include sports such as running, exercising, playing tennis and could also include such actions as playing instruments, talking nature walks and even primping and prepping our bodies for the day by doing hair, makeup or dressing.

Given that it has only been in the past decade of my own life that I've become interested in physical activities like running and yoga, I was keenly aware that some of my students may not be involved in team sports and might, as a result, feel they had nothing about which to write. I wanted to stress that we all have a connection to our bodies and hoped my students would accept my open invitation to take the prompt in the direction they felt adequately addressed their body movements, as uniquely situated as each body from which they sprang. No matter the direction, I asked my students to consider questions such as, "How does your body express itself in these activities? How do your body and mind work together? Or, how do your thinking and movement fit together in these activities? Can you give specific examples (take time to detail them)? How might your body sometimes lead your mind in those activities (my favorite example here is how we often just drive without thinking and wonder later how we ever got to our destination). You should also think about what have you learned about your body and its expression from these activities. As you re-read your writing here, what have you not thought about before about being an active body-mind that this blog is making you explore?"

Not surprisingly, the most active athletes in the class relished the opportunity to discuss their activities and kinesthetic knowledge for this blog. And what surprised me the most was that so many of my students were involved in university teams as well as intramural sports. Others were similarly committed to playing instruments or continuing activities, such as running or swimming, performed as part of a high school team, which remained a crucial aspect of my students' identities. Even if they did not compete at the university level on structured teams, my students described their physical activities as central parts of themselves and their weekly schedules. Everyone agreed that this blog was the easiest to write because it was the closest to their daily experiences and allowed them to share bits of themselves that would normally remain hidden in a writing class.

Lacy, a student swimmer showed a great level of proprioception in her second body blog response:

> Nothing beats the feeling of my muscles working, pulling deep into the water, propelling me forward. The complete physical aspect of the sport is so enticing to me when my brain feels like it might explode. However, swimming is not only a physical sport, but it is a mental sport as well. Swimmers have to be totally focused, especially in practice. Practice is the time to think about the technicalities of the stroke. "Is my streamline tight enough?" "Are my elbows high enough to catch the maximum amount of water?" "Am I kicking the right distance off the wall to maximize my momentum from the turn?

For Lacy, the physical strength necessary to succeed at this water sport must be accompanied by a great body awareness, so great that she must rely on her body's intelligence to maximize her winning potential, which comes down to fractions of a second as she explains later in the same response. Lacy's description nicely points to the ways she uses a version of the embodied imagination to feel her body's spatial positioning: only by learning how her arms feel and which muscles tighten can she sense how high her elbows are when she is in the water. Mindfulness of her body and its placement and desires is necessary for her success as a swimmer, and she can only achieve this level of awareness when she sees herself as a whole piece, as body and brain working together to achieve future goals and embrace present realities. Lacy's classmate, Will, a golfer, describes a similar experience of embodied awareness on the green:

> I play golf very often, as much as six days a week during the summer weather permitting. My body has the movements of my golf swing deeply engrained. However I often make minor changes or tweaks to my golf swing as needed to improve it or put it back into place if pieces have moved around a bit …. Pieces are never in exactly the same place, as many things can affect the way you set up to the ball. And any change in the set up will change the swing. I have found that even the clothes I wear can affect the way I set up. For example, I have discovered that I more easily get into proper set up position if I wear pants compared to when I wear shorts. My theory is that the pants give me the feeling of having a slightly lower center of gravity. But if my body and mind weren't connected, I would never remember from day to day how to hit the ball …. I am trying to connect my body and mind in golf more by trying to be better able to visualize my swing and learn to play more by feel and instinct, which is hard to do when you are given all this time to think about what you are going to do before you do it.

This response is exemplary in its detailed description of how this student's body and mind work together when playing golf, which is why I quote it at length. The way Will works toward the importance of visualization for his sport and how he pins the successful expression of his swing on the integration of his physical body and mental body are examples of insights I hoped some students might stumble upon in these blogs. Will not only imagines himself as an integrated whole as a golfer, which will hopefully encourage a transfer of meaning so he will eventually see himself as a writing body, but he also articulates a version of the embodied imagination I proposed in my introduction and expanded in the last chapter.

Will continues to describe his attitude toward change as a competitive golfer on the university team. He notes particularly the ways imagining changes and differences *as* embodied, as impacted by materiality and rooted in the real, gives him a freedom of expression he cannot capture solely in language:

> When making changes [to my swing], I have discovered it's easier to make a visual of the change and feel it compared to trying to put it into words. Our bodies have a harder time interpreting words than images and feelings of movement. But what is maybe the most important thing in golf is making sure your body and mind are aimed at the same target. For example, if your body is aimed the pond, but you are thinking about the green left of the pond, chances are you are going to hit the ball towards the pond …. This really makes me wonder how the mind-body connection is present in all activities.

For Will, the imagination is situated quite literally in the body and impacted by it. As he states, his swing is shaped by his body's positioning, no matter where he hopes the ball will land. In this way, he knows to be sensitive to his flesh and to respect his sport's engagement of *both* his body and mind. Mindless fragmentation of his being is detrimental to his success as a golfer and, he will soon learn, to his effectiveness as a writer. So perceptive about his remarks is his focus on how feelings and sensory images are just as meaningful in the process of his practice as fully-formed verbal thoughts and words. This student is already versed in the ways that imagining ourselves as embodied necessitates an understanding of situated thinking and feeling as mutually constitutive and reinforcing. Will testifies to the ways the body as signifier cannot exhaust the meaning of materiality which exceeds even language.

Of course, not all students' prior experiences lend for such for such easy transfer. For some students, the body-mind connection is much more troubled at first and presents a confusing paradox. Caleb states that

> [As a musician and guitarist] I guess I can never really be one hundred percent certain if it is in fact my mind telling my body what to do because sometimes I feel like my body has a mind of its own. Wow, I find it ironic the way I just worded that because it seems to have disproved my point. Everything is much more complicated than people would think things to be …. When I hear a song I log it mentally in my head and then I pick up my guitar and start playing. Sure, it takes a few tries for me to get a song down correctly, but I learn to play it pretty fast and I haven't forgotten a song that I learned yet. My fingers just happen to go to the right place

> at the right time and it works. I think it's something that happens unconsciously at first, and then I realize what is going on and I work with it.

Caleb, a guitarist, understands on a felt level that his body is at work in his learning to play new songs, as his "fingers just happen to go to the right place," but he still seems disconnected from the process. While he might recognize his body as an epistemic origin, he doesn't have the conceptual maps to understand how this might work, likely because our learning culture often doesn't provide these. As a result, Caleb "feel[s] like [his] body has a mind of its own," and he says he doesn't understand this mind—even when he follows it after a while, after realizing "what is going on" as his fingers move on his guitar strings. This description is fascinating for its revelation of how much body awareness and attentiveness to his corporeal orientation could help Caleb unify his fingers' energy and intelligence with his mind's desire to learn a new song. With mindfulness of his body, Caleb might be able to understand the playing of music and the composing of writing from a new, contemplative and visceral perspective. And this might help him appreciate why his body moves in unpredictable ways at times:

> Unfortunately, I feel like the body, even though it is connected to the mind, acts on its own sometimes. I think that some of the time the body reacts to things before the mind comprehends what is going on. For example, when I'm bored in a class or in anything my body shows that boredom even when my brain knows that I shouldn't be slouching or anything. My body moves on its own even if I tell it not to and to pay attention. Things happen that I can't control sometimes …. [My body] moves in ways that I can't understand, yet it also helps me in my music and in other areas. Having the two connected is better than having them as separates.

Caleb's continued meditation on the body reminds me of the first lessons I learned in my yoga classes about respecting the body by asking less for control over it. Exchanging connection for control helps us to channel the body's energies in pleasing and productive ways, eliminating the frustration we might otherwise feel. While Caleb knows such connection is ideal from his experiences playing, he is unsure how to facilitate it and sees his body as disruptive in more formal learning environments, beyond the limits of his control. Of course, we may begin to wonder if this is more a result of restrictive learning environments that are not guided by embodied-contemplative educational principles which would have students learning how meaning is made with and through the body, by focusing its energies.

After asking for the first two blogs and noting in my students' responses equal measures of understanding and confusion, I then asked students to bring together any insights they might have made in the process of completing this assignment and to forward any interesting, new questions, bringing both to bear on their writing. The third body blog's guiding question was, "How can you become a better writing by using body-mind skill sets you already have?" I explained to students that the blogs were meant to get them thinking about how their bodies might play a larger part in our thinking and expression than we normally realize. By building off the last set of responses, I wanted them to analyze the irony of imagining themselves as bodies during certain activities in which they were encouraged to see themselves of a whole, integrated piece but not during others, such as writing.

I didn't want students to begin to reify their bodies or account for every movement in the writing process as bodily; rather, I wanted them to discover the agency of their writing bodies in partnership to their minds, to see their intelligence as a union of both. In all, the final blog entry asked students to reflect on the ways the body and the mind are connected in interesting, inter-related and interdependent ways. Building on the guiding question, the full, detailed description for this blog read: "To finish your final installment, bring your insights from the first two blogs together. Read them over and revisit your thoughts and feelings. Discuss your initial responses in the first two installments. Anything you'd change now? Any new insights you'd like to bring to bear on them? Think specifically about the body-mind awareness you may have discussed in blog two in terms of your physical activities. How could you draw on this awareness to become a better writer? Can you apply some of the same techniques, say, that make you a good swimmer or baseball player, etc., to your writing process? Be specific and give examples/details. Can you learn anything about listening to your body as you write, either metaphorically (ie., in terms of calling upon personal experiences in essays) or literally (ie., in terms of endurance)? How you might bring more awareness to the process of writing? What parallels can you make? Where do the two not seem to fit? Where are there tensions and why might they exist? What may you realize now that you've completed the body blog that you didn't before?"

An overriding theme in students' responses to this final comparison of body blog installations one and two is that of body appreciation and a budding corporeal awareness. To quote Nikki, the student I open this interchapter with, is to echo the rest: "I always believed in the concept of the body being far less important than the mind. But after some thought about the subject, I have come to the realization that the body and mind are equally as important in making up an individual ... and that affects my writing." That these blogs helped students like Nikki begin to think of themselves holistically, as one piece, was crucial in their beginning learning process for our class. Not only would they appreciate the lessons of our units on disability, eating, body image and identity more from this point on, but they would now be ready to investigate the physicality of the writing process through other embodied acts such as yoga. While obviously not the final step in accepting themselves as writing bodies, my students were now questioning the ways they saw writing as "mind work" and why they divided this kind of work from body work. They began to wonder with renewed appreciation the ways their other classes locked their bodies out. And, they began to inquire how this new knowledge could change their experiences of the writing process and the ways they approached writing assignments from this point onward.

For instance, Lacey, the swimmer, found new meaning in the drafting process; for her, understanding her writing body as a viable player in the meaning-making process meant respecting the ways that body-based skills take time to develop. She notes, "I really think that now I should begin my assignments when I get them assigned because I feel that I will now need to revise many of my papers and writings before they are due and that time is limited if I begin the assignment the day or night before." Instead of procrastination, Lacey believes she should start to apply her "swimming stamina of being able to be focused on one goal" even when the finish line is nowhere in sight because her "body is at stake." Given that we all want our students to spend more time and effort in their writing and to take their drafts through multiple, global revisions, this is an important discovery this student may not have made if she weren't invited to apply the body skills and knowledge she already has to the writing process, helping her begin a process of demystification that encouraged motivation. Not to be overlooked is the way reconceptualizing the writing process as visceral helps such students actively engage their bodies in it rather than trying to ignore them, which may prove to be distracting. Because she had previously conceptualized writing as a process distinct from swimming, Lacy noted, in fact, that when "normally when engaged in writing, my body is tired and bored." Learning to respect her body and investigate why it was bored (in part because it was ignored) helped this student create new writing rituals that resulted in less painful writing sessions and recognize the need to give himself ample time for writing breaks, cutting through her habitual procrastination.

This student notes that using this "swimming stamina" will allow her to apply a new measure of focus to her writing as well. Lacy states, "That way when I write I am only focused on the subject of the paper and not who is on Facebook or who just texted me. For example during a swim race I rarely ever think about anything except my stroke, turns, and winning the race or beating my most current time." Noting as well the overwhelming nature of being constantly surrounded by technological distractions as he wrote, another student, Steve, agreed that he learned through the blogs that slowing down his writing process would help promote focus and increase the quality of his writing in turn. Steve claimed he could apply lessons of focus and interconnection to his writing, drawn from his experiences playing baseball. Steve reflects,

> One principle I can maybe apply to better my writing is to slow down. As I mentioned in my earlier blog, when I'm playing well in baseball (or any other sport for that matter), everything seems to slow down for me. I feel like I have more time to react, and therefore am able to better affect my results .... If I were somehow able to slow my mind down and pick what minor details are important, while maintaining focus on the larger issue, I feel like I could improve my writing significantly. Often I am too straight to the point, and I rush to get down my ideas and prove my thesis. I need to slow things down, like I do in baseball, and put some of the smaller things that I admire into my writing.

Steve might be hinting at the ways our minds and bodies work together in what has been called physiological coherence. In activities like sports and many disciplines of contemplation like meditation, the body, heart, brain and nervous system synchronize with one another, which can lead to improved attention often perceived as a slowing down of time and described as being "in the zone." At these times of body-mind harmony, students may experience increased performance and a decrease of stress and anxiety because of a "regular heart rhythm, decreased sympathetic nervous system activation and increased parasympathetic activity and increased heart-brain synchronized (the brain's alpha rhythms becomes more synchronized to the heartbeat) (Schooner & Kelso, 1988; Tiller, McCraty & Atkinson, 1996; quoted in Hart, 2004, p. 31).[10] This knowledge can be applied to the reverse as well. That is, when students don't feel this kind of physiological coherence, they might take a writing break in order to later return to the writing process later with a refocused mind—a valuable lesson. Mary vocalized this insight: "When you write, you can also listen to your body by learning when you're tired. Writing when your body and brain are tired is a waste because your work will come out sloppy and rushed. When I write and become tired or sick of writing, my hand or foot will begin to tap. If I know my body well enough, I can take this as a sign to take a break and finish my writing at another time." This is a lesson of learning to work *with* as opposed to attempting to overwrite the body's intelligence and of being mindful of our embodied feelings in the present moment, which is the practice of mindfulness. In their movement toward imagining themselves as writing bodies, students work toward more reflective and less reflexive understandings and negotiations of the writing process.

Finally, some students noted that their bodies could become sources of inspiration and energy for the writing process, drawing off the idea that the physical writing body can provide shape to writing through feeling and the motivation to write. Jamie, challenging her previous belief that her body has no place in her writing so that to accommodate it would surely "do her in" noted, "Often times when you are assigned a writing assignment about an event in your life, you need just look at your scars for reminders on what to write about." In her later blogs, Jamie became interested in the ways emotion could be seen as a link to the invention state of writing, giving her an impetus to write: "In addition, I could also draw on the energy I get when I am feeling upset, angry, or stressed into writing. I would normally take this energy into a physical activity and feel like I could achieve the impossible because my mind just went through the motions of the activity … .my body goes hand in hand with my emotions." It is no coincidence that students like Jamie are articulating a premise of contemplative pedagogy, or the need to respect the visceral nature of feeling and the ways the heart can be a bridge to the mind and body.

While more a start than an end, these body blogs asked students to investigate seriously their writing identities and personas as necessarily embodied. They gave my students a foundational understanding of what it means to write aware of both body and mind and how a focus on self-examination and awareness can help increase their productivity and enjoyment of the writing process. As students crossed the threshold of knowing they *have* a body to becoming aware of *how* that body impacts the meaning they make in their writing, the made adjustments to their writing processes in order to respect their flesh. They began seeing themselves as writing yogis who enacted the principles of the embodied imagination.

BODY BLOGS IN CONTEXT

Through their body blogs, my students began their journey to take on new understandings of themselves as writing yogis. To further exercise their embodied imaginations, we also read articles that acknowledged the importance of incorporating embodied experience as evidence into our writing, a common feature of contemplative learning which adds attention to personal presence and social transformation along with subject matter knowledge and rational empiricism. For example, we read Linda Brodkey's Writing on the Bias to talk about how our writing is "biased" by our experiences and ideas even when we don't use the word, "I," directly. Brodkey becomes a way for students to understand the basics of situated knowledge, or the ways their social and material locatedness shapes the meaning they write themselves to. She also helps me frame these lessons for transfer, so students understand that what they are learning in my classroom are lessons about the situatedness of knowledge claims and, therefore, of writing. They begin to understand that there is something fundamental about these ways of thinking about knowledge in all their classes across the many discourse communities they must join as students—even if stylistic functions of writing (as a means to build knowledge) acceptable in my class are not similarly so in their science or engineering classes. Putting Brodkey in play with our own quest to unveil the physical aspects of writing helps them see how the body becomes a marker for the personal in their writings. Because they've often questioned the ability to gain authority in their writing by simply leaving out personal markers like, "in my opinion" or first-person pronouns, generally, my students relate to Brodkey:

> Brodkey wants her reader to see that ... sometimes the rules [of academic writing] need to be broken. I began to think about how much this was true, that it is important to deviate sometimes in order to explore new terrain to not only be successful in writing but in other aspects of life as well .... I have had a very successful golfing career because I broke some of the rules, tried new things, and was able to learn from them—and this [risk-taking] was the main reason in my growing as a writer this semester.

The personal and the body collide and mingle in this response. Students, as this example shows, begin to apply their knowledge of other body skills to the writing process, giving them a store of information based on the physical skills they import into my class, like golf. When put into embodied dialogue with what they know and love, suddenly writing becomes a physical process much like their other activities, allowing this student, in particular, to apply the lessons of risk-taking she originally learned on the green to her writing process and the meaning it generates. The degree to which this kind of transfer makes writing more accessible for our students cannot be overstated. Either can the ways my student insists on developing a habit of taking risks because of this transfer, which opens her up for failure but also for greater success.

To advance these insights, we read articles by Nancy Sommers on how writing can happen while "standing," away from the computer,[11] while cooking or completing other daily tasks. Writing doesn't just move us, it moves, my students learn as they open and expand their definitions of the writing process to include the body. These articles make writing seem real to my students because they help demystify the process. The myth of sitting down to a computer allowing words to spill out from the fountain of genius is challenged, and students seem relieved. Despite the fact that the myth has never been the reality of their writing experiences to date, they often import these whimsical views of writing to my class. Anne Lamott's (2005) Shitty First Drafts helps to break this stereotype too. And, Natalie Goldberg's discussion of freewriting in Writing Down the Bones (2005) as a way to get your body to convince your mind to generate ideas helps students realize they don't have to wait for their minds to do the leading; that their bodies can help them reach their writing goals too. We also read Joanne Cavanaugh Simpson's anthologized article, Multitasking State of Mind (2009), which suggests that college teachers must help students learn to overcome the multitasking minds they've had no choice but to develop in our technologically-demanding world. The article looks for possible tools to achieve a transformation of mindless students into mindful ones and ends with the idea that bringing in a yoga teacher to our classrooms might be a good place to start. I tell my students that is exactly what we are going to do, of course. By this time, students are generally intrigued and ready to experiment with yoga—even if they are still nervous. In the next two interchapters, I explore how I introduce students to a yoga-writing practice, scaffolded by our body blogs. In the following chapter, I take time to explore first why feminist contemplative pedagogies give meaning to students' explorations of embodiment in ways other pedagogies cannot as fruitfully explain or uphold.

CHAPTER TWO: PERSONAL PRESENCE, EMBODIED EMPIRICISM AND RESONANCE IN CONTEMPLATIVE WRITING

> We teach in a culture that simultaneously obsesses about and disregards bodies and in an academic culture that still views teachers and students as 'minds' and 'intellects' only .... Our theories of pedagogy cannot afford to neglect the dancing bodies in our classrooms.
> —Tina Kazan, Dancing Bodies in the Classroom

Tina Kazan's reevaluation of "dancing bodies" in my epigraph is rooted in her visceral experience as a body who navigates the pedagogical spaces of both ballrooms and writing classrooms. Kazan bridges her embodied experiences as a writing teacher to hers as a student of ballroom dancing in order to illuminate how all writing teachers are dually implicated in a process of reading bodies and—because we maintain positions of power in the classroom however much we attempt to eschew our authority—sanctioning them. Like the dance instructor who (mistakenly) reads Kazan and her lesbian friend as a couple but cannot transcend the heteronormative ballroom dancing language on which she relies, teachers sanction how bodies are allowed to speak in the classroom. Sanctioning takes place via the ways teachers literally see the bodies before them and the corresponding ways they gesture to bodies in language.

Here, the eye confers location and space to the process of situating and reading embodied others. Indeed, Kazan uses Mikhail Bakhtin's theory of the "surplus of seeing," or the idea that because each body is necessarily opaque to itself, can literally only see outward, to argue for the relationality of bodies to each other and the need to understand situatedness as stemming literally from the point of view of the fleshy body. Understanding situatedness as arising not just from discursive placement but also from the "situated nature of perspective" (Kazan, 2005, p. 385) invites an understanding of how composition teachers "teach writers, bodies who aspire to write" (Kazan, 2005, p. 392). In ways akin to contemplative writing pedagogy, Kazan defines the process of (teaching) writing as one that always already involves the body and therefore as one that could be strengthened if explicit attention were paid to material relations in teaching and learning.

In sharp contrast to Kazan's concept of dancing-writing bodies is what Worsham has termed the "wild subject," the prevalent constructivist concept used to denote the writing subject in composition studies (2001, p. 247). Worsham's term highlights a state of detachment that makes the subject unrestrained or "wild," as it is permitted and encouraged to rise above its body. The wild subject is a rhetorical subject, to be sure, making it highly useful for analysis, but this picture of subjectivity has come at the cost of valuing materiality in the ways both Worsham and Kazan hope we might. When given space in language as a subject and not approached as a writing body, the writer remains rhetorical because she can transcend her material composition, placing value on her consciousness over and above (as removable) from her flesh.[12] As this hierarchy is normalized in our pedagogical and professional writing, it follows that it becomes part of the hidden curriculum, or as Worsham might say, part of the dominant pedagogy, we teach our students. We need only to look as far as the students discussed in Interchapter One to see the consequences of this dominant pedagogy. Students there couldn't recognize the ironies of seeing writing only in terms of thinking, even when their bodies screamed for attention, because they were so well schooled to rise above the gross body when attending to matters of the mind. In dominant schooling systems, it is difficult to affirm the importance of the material relations between writing bodies, a difficulty my students had to confront in their body blogs outlined there.

This difficulty is what Kazan hopes to address. Her article can be placed within a new wave of scholarship on what might be called "embodied writing pedagogy" which has begun to restore focus on the individual writer as a means of reclaiming her materiality. Despite developing interest in materiality (Hawhee, Fleckenstein) and positionality (Kazan), however, embodied writing remains a somewhat scattered approach. I argue in this chapter that contemplative writing represents a more sustainable and interdisciplinary (and, therefore, writing-across-the-curriculum friendly) learning approach and praxis that captures the importance of our felt experiences without denying the responsibility of critically investigating our embodiment and connecting with others in ways responsible to our (and their) flesh.

As previous chapters have illustrated, I seek to maximize the coherence between the feminist and the contemplative in my work. Giving contemplative writing studies a feminist edge through the feminist epistemology theorized by

Haraway, in particular, adds to its strengths and provides a different method of knowing for our field—and, therein, a different picture of subjectivity. The union also generates a new means of writing instruction, what I've been referring to as feminist contemplative writing pedagogy. If my last chapter explored how a writing subject might reconnect her "wild" mind with her organic, intelligent body by understanding herself as a writing yogi, a body-heart-mind, then this chapter will follow the consequences of this shift for the meaning-making process of writing itself and the knowledge construction that occurs as a result of this process; both are consciously located within their material contexts in contemplative pedagogy. Rather than valuing third-person knowing to the effect of erasing the knower's body, contemplative pedagogies work to better understand the dynamics of first-person knowing and seek to find resonance between varied sources of embodied, felt knowledge. They forward a picture of knowing as advanced by the skill of embodied imagining, as outlined in my introduction.

This is a view of knowledge as local and embodied that contemporary cognitive neuroscience has begun to validate. Neurophenomenology, a new, integrative branch of neuroscience, has sought to theorize consciousness from a paradigm of embodiment. Coined by the late scientist Francisco Varela, neurophenomenology argues for an enactive or embedded approach to cognition, one that seeks to position experience as embodied and intersubjective and to understand cognition as including factors such as the body and the world and not just the brain (Rudrauf, Lutz, Cosmelli, Lachaux, & Le Van Quyen, 2003, p. 33). Two main consequences of this scientific approach include a valuation of our flesh, now seen as "the root of our experience" as well as a valorization of first-person, subjective knowledge (Rudrauf et al., 2003, pp. 33; 37). These reclamations of the individual have recently led Cooper to argue that neurophenomenology can help us navigate responsible rhetorical agency (2011, p. 420). As intimately tied to neuroscience, contemplative pedagogy presents us with the opportunity to explore these developments within our field, giving us new means to explore the embodied and experiential nature of writing and writers, and Haraway gives us a feminist topos from which to do this work.

Contemplative embodiment might yet remain an underexplored paradigm for knowing and writing in our field (though not others), but the experiential has a long history within our scholarship: most notably, through its entanglement with expressivist approaches. As a learning methodology geared to the whole person, it's (too) easy to read contemplative pedagogy as nouveau-expressivism. Expressivism, understood as a pedagogy of "the personal," shares with contemplative writing pedagogy a desire to centrally locate the writer and to validate her experiences. The advantage of such a reading is its effect: how the contemplative is thusly brought into the historical fold of composition studies and into dialogue with existing approaches to the personal and the experiential. The disadvantage is that to engage with expressivism at all is to risk assuming its massive emotional and historical baggage. However, dialoguing contemplative pedagogical approaches with others more established in our field is important work if we hope to establish a lasting place for the contemplative in our theory and practice—exactly why I briefly go to expressivist theory in the pages that follow. Even so, while the dialogue is useful, the comparison between these two pedagogical approaches reveals more crucial differences than similarities. Contemplative writing pedagogy, with its focus on lived, social responsibility and embodied situatedness doesn't entertain expressivism's perceived solipsism or its essentialist conception of the autonomous self understood outside of the community; it exchanges the closed system of meaning within Romanticism for more worldly, connected systems within contemplative theory, such as the Eastern philosophies of yoga, which balance inner- and outer-directedness.

Contemplative writing reanimates the personal by keeping the embodied presence of the writer visible at all times while simultaneously attending to a corporeal-cultural situatedness that accounts for resonant connections with embodied others and a larger material world of which we are a part. Additionally, contemplative pedagogies expand our learning approaches to include:

- "an *epistemology of presence* that moves past conditioned habits of mind to stay awake in the here and now.
- a *pedagogy of resonance* that shapes our graciousness and spaciousness toward meeting and receiving the world nondefensively.
- a *more intimate and integral empiricism* that includes in the consideration of the question a reflection on ourselves and on the question itself" (Hart, 2008, p. 237).

All together, these approaches and corresponding skills, outlined by contemplative educator Hart, assert the materiality of the knower, of knowledge and of the meaning-making process of writing. With Hart, I approach contemplative pedagogy through the three lenses of presence, resonance and embodied-connected empiricism by asking three corollary questions, pertinent to the field of rhetoric and composition studies, in particular:

- *Presence:* How do we understand the "personal" in written texts and in relation to the embodied writer in feminist contemplative writing pedagogy? How exactly do we validate her presence and agency?
- *Resonance:* How might the contemplative writer mindfully approach and receive her attachments and connections to the world of matter, including her physical environments, her material writing process and

habits and other bodies in the world?
- *Embodied Empiricism:* While maintaining the need for outer-directedness, how can we simultaneously validate lived experience as a form of local knowledge and a valuable source of evidence for writing produced within contemplative pedagogies?

In what follows, I bring these three queries of contemplative learning to bear on our field by exploring the cost of denying the writing body as an epistemic origin and by addressing the benefits of situating the *person* and her experiences at the center of our theories of writing within contemplative pedagogy.

THE PRESENCE OF THE PERSON(AL)

Advocate of embodied writing Hindman uses an expressivist notion of the personal subject to drive her essay, Making Writing Matter: Using "The Personal" to Recover[y] an Essential[ist] Tension in Academic Discourse. She highlights for me both the strengths of an epistemology of presence as well as the reasons why expressivist paradigms cannot fully support the requisite attention to matter. In her essay, Hindman attempts to show how the authority of the expressivist personal self must be reclaimed for embodied rhetorics. Hindman does not suggest we naively return to any essentialized notions of the self that are not aware of our social or linguistic construction—this is an attachment she does not want to lose. Rather, Hindman notes that we need to better hold tension between an expressive, personal self and a cultural, socially-constructed self in order to attend to our materiality as writers (2001, p. 89). Essentially, she argues for a double gesture, claiming that neither subject position alone will work; our attempt to move *from* one *to* another evades the real issue of our corporeality. Because she is interested in reclaiming the material person behind the personal, Hindman outlines the consequences of adopting a contemplative approach to composing, one that reattaches the corporeal presence of the writer to her writing.

To be attentive to matter, Hindman advocates writing our experiences and bodies into our prose as impetus and evidence for our arguments. In this way, our writing becomes personal, or evidentially full of its fleshy author. It's the claiming and self-awareness of this fullness—a fullness that upends a habitual tendency to write over the material—that contemplative pedagogy calls presence. Using her experience to navigate the theoretically thorny issue of subjectivity, Hindman's main objective is to consider "how [her] personal experience with alcoholism and with the discourse of recovery demonstrates to [her] the futility—indeed, the conceit—of trying to dispel the tension between competing versions of how the self is constructed" (2001, p. 92). Hindman believes that holding onto the expressivist self, because it accounts for personal experience, will invite the body that poststructuralist constructivism has overwritten back "in," allowing it to count in our writerly quest for understanding and meaning. The expressivist self gives Hindman hope for reclaiming presence.

While I agree with the spirit of Hindman's struggle, another way of looking at her attempt to resolve expressivist and constructivist notions of subjectivity with each other is to see both as fatally flawed. To follow Hindman, we must see our field as coalescing still around two pedagogical touchstones, that of expressivism and constructivism. That's an argument I don't take on here, since many others have, but I do want to address the irony of this pedagogical configuration: it hides the implicit agreement between these two approaches that we earn presence as writers by *transcending* our flesh, not mindfully claiming it. A careful look at some foundational texts that outline the differences of these approaches shows how the Western tradition of downplaying the body for the mind is evidenced in contemporary constructivist and expressivist pedagogies as *both* work to detach us from the materiality of our lived bodies and experiences. If critical constructivism promises transcendence from the body through theories of discursive production wherein the subject is always interpolated by a discourse that precedes it, an essentialist-leaning expressivism[13] does no better as it promises transcendence through an individual mind that can rise above its social environment as well as the limitations of the body (Crick, 2003, p. 257), negating the role of materiality. If nature, and the body in turn, can never be known in itself because culture is always mediating it, then nature is just another word for culture, and our only agency lies in constructivist narratives (Berlin, 2003, p. 76). In both, the only presence writers can fully claim is linguistic.

Bordo names this kind of faith in the rhetoric of linguistic construction to make us "present" the "epistemological fantasy of *becoming* multiplicity" (1993, p. 145). It is this dream of limitless multiplicity and rhetoricity that Hindman argues against, which is why she places more—perhaps too much—hope in the material attachments of expressivism. For her, constructivist approaches lose the real, even biological ways her body is already an alcoholic prior to the discursive tag and the corresponding rhetoric surrounding this label. Denied matter(ing), the body has no real presence in this dominant pedagogical approach; it becomes the "no body" of postmodernism that Bordo challenges.

Offering something akin to a Platonic "fantasy of authenticity," expressivism unfortunately gets us no closer to claiming the material presence of the writer despite Hindman's hope that it might. Expressivist attention to the self has been thoroughly critiqued for forwarding a romantic notion of the mind/soul because this is an essentialist view of the subject; this view provides the tension Hindman wants in her double gesture. Yet from the perspective of the contemplative, expressivist subjectivity is problematic because it forwards a disembodied notion of the self as reducible to the free floating mind/soul. Despite their focus on experience, expressivists have not only promoted ideas of students rising above the collective in order to express an ineffable personal self, they have also equated this self with the individual's mind, ignoring the weight of corporeality. A contemplative-minded fullness of presence is denied: the expressivist mind/soul is often identified *as* the person(al), so that the concrete body becomes a mere fleshy vehicle for the psyche and not an origin of presence for our writing and identity.

The expressive transcendent mind as divorceable from the flesh is a conception that enforces the separation of a consciousness from the body that acts primarily as a vehicle and/or extension of its internal thoughts. In turn, experience is emptied of its materiality, valued as an effect or a memory contained by the intellect and as fodder for personal reflection. Elbow's classic "movies of the mind" metaphor highlights the way meaning in expressivist epistemology is often seen as removed from the experiencing body. Elbow locates meaning in the individual's consciousness with his "movies of the mind:"

> Meaning is like movies inside the head. I've got movies in my head. I want to put them inside yours. Only I can't do that because our heads are opaque. All I can do is try to be clever about sending you a sound track and hope I've done it in such a way as to make you construct the right movies in your head. (1973, p. 152)

In this iconic Western formulation, meaning from experience is something shaped by the mind and remains something that wishes to "get out" through language expression. Like in constructivist pedagogy, presence remains linguistic not material. On both accounts, thoughts exist unchained to bodies. Enacted through our writing, the "I" of expressivist personal writing seems to be more an individual mind's expression of itself than an embodied "I" that expresses the real presence of a writing body, how we might approach the personal within feminist-contemplative writing pedagogy.

Elbow's "movies of the mind" may be an older configuration of expressivist meaning making systems, which expand beyond Elbow himself, but it remains a classic feature of expressivist thinking. Earlier talk of "movies of the mind" has now shifted to talk of language itself, in part due to contemporary efforts to bring this pedagogy in dialogue with social constructionist pedagogy. Developing what has been called social expressivism (Gradin), compositionists such as Ann Berthoff have moved expressivist meaning into the paradigm of social constructionism. Yet, new versions are still rooted in a basic, untenable relationship to matter that overwrites it with language, even if they now find meaning in the interaction of a social language and the individual psyche and not the latter alone. Berthoff's discussion of how meaning is made in this relational process may mediate tension between the individual and the cultural, but it does little to alleviate tension between the body and mind: "By naming the world, we hold images in mind; we remember; we can return to our experience and reflect on it. In reflecting, we can change, we can transform, we can envisage. Language thus becomes the very type of social activity by which we might move towards changing our lives" (Berthoff p. 751; quoted in Gradin, 1995, p. 115). Her explanation shows how social expressivism still supports a devaluation of matter by advancing a dichotomy between body and mind that draws on the immaterialism of both traditional expressivism and constructivism. Echoing back to Elbow's movies of the mind, the embodiment of experience in Berthoff's explanation seems to matter much less, if at all, than the way language is used to shape it or memory is used to store/ configure it. Expressivism remains largely disembodied—surprising for a pedagogy based in experience.

As Berthoff shows, the power of personal experience in classic and contemporary expressivism rests neither with having the experience nor the physicality of our meaning making in writing; instead it rests with the power of naming or intellectualizing experience through language. Contemplative pedagogy would agree that naming experience is indeed a shaping activity, an important one at that, but would argue that it isn't the end, or isn't exhaustive of meaning and that we mustn't ignore the fullness of embodied presence. Whether viewed through classic formations or new ones indebted to constructionist understandings of the self as socially written through language, expressivism empties experience of its material connection—why updated notions of the personal plucked from expressivist theory have not yet claimed the material body's presence. Extending Berthoff's work in new directions, Candace Spigelman seems to recognize this dilemma. She attempts to move the personal out from the jurisdiction of expressivism in order to give it viability and show how it can be a social concept and not just a synonym for the psyche. In *Personally Speaking*, her book-length treatment of this complex term, Spigelman states, the "personal involves a particular way of conveying information that seems to represent an autonomous writer's unmediated reflection on his or her 'authentic' lived experience" (2004, p. 30). This is the essence of the critique against expressivist pedagogy. Her effort in reclaiming the personal is to "detach" it from these limited conceptions by understanding it instead as a rhetorical construct, as fully mediated by a social language (2004, p. 30). Spigelman's move to rhetoricize the personal is one that could finally bring it under the postmodern rubric by questioning its autonomy and the "free" or "private" space this concept seems to invite.

Spigelman does realize that such a move necessarily cuts the personal away from the fabric of the material. But, she is committed to rhetoricizing the personal in order to give it new viability, so this author notes her choice to table a discussion of materiality (2004, p. 33). She doesn't linger over corporeality lost in her model because she sees no way of asserting material presence without engaging in the binary between matter and discourse and ultimately supporting one term over the other. In refusing to engage the complexity, however, Spigelman may implicate herself in those discussions of materiality she claims to find inherently reductive (2004, p. 33). Her concern over binaries, along with the "anxiety" (2004, p. 60) that she claims accompanies the debate over the personal, leads her to see this epistemological term as a representative label within her pedagogy, valued for the space in language it guarantees. This semiotic space allows her to reassert the academic value of personal writing within a field turned largely constructivist; personal writing as argument is her focus. But, embracing the personal as more than a discursive label neither means necessarily unmooring it from its anchorage in the body nor does attention to materiality need to be reductive. In a professional environment that has moved closer to addressing the importance of the material than it had when Spigelman was writing, we have more options than this.

Offering a hopeful alternative, feminist contemplative writing pedagogy restores our focus on experience while attending to the personal body not as ineffable but as embedded and present. The body is what gives us an anchor through "subjective factual truth while the mind generat[es] imaginative ideas" (Iyengar, 2005, p. 162). Here, the embodied imagination shapes experience into knowledge by helping to construct meaning and to stretch it in new directions. Contemplative practices like *asana* teach writers the skill of embodied imagining, or how to balance having the experience with processing it because "it is the precise, thorough measuring and adjustment of a pose [or action], bringing balance, stability and equal extension everywhere that hones this faculty of discrimination …. Intelligence … becomes muscular"; imagination becomes embodied (Iyengar, 2005, pp. 162-163). Indeed, the agency of the writing yogi who exercises her embodied imagination is tied up with her ability to put thoughts into action: *tapas*, such as the physical action of *asana*, is key to embody the imagination and "transfor[m] the shapes of mind into reality" (Iyengar, 2005, p. 157).

This is a discerning action, one that moves mindfully in directions dictated by our intentions and not reactive habit. Actions and agency, therefore, rest on presence in contemplative writing pedagogy.

MATERIAL RESONANCE THROUGH PERSONAL PRESENCE

In contemplative practice, learning to be fully present (presence) is a practice mastered by learning to find our center as well as to recognize our integration within a larger world of material others (resonance). The yogi practices moving meditations, *asana*, and breathing meditations, *pranayama*, to develop her skills as an embodied imaginer. These practices help her to experience herself holistically as mind, physical body and emotional body and to see herself as embedded within a larger community through which she finds resonance by virtue of her shared materiality. Similarly, within feminist contemplative writing pedagogy, a fullness of personal presence must include both the social and the material. Because presence is both embodied and enacted, it is a skill that can be developed by contemplative writing and learning practices which train writers to both respect their inner lives and (in doing so) their connection to an external world that enfolds them. The heuristic for this kind of writing-learning is attachment. That is, the contemplative relates the embodied personal and the culturally enacted, *which come together under the full rubric of embodiment*, and requires us to leave behind both the wild subject of postmodernism as well as the personal subjectivity embraced by early expressivism. It is no coincidence that the contemplative leads us to a fuller, more incorporative understanding of the personal by way of its emphasis on resonance.

Haraway theorizes a notion of the personal that presents the possibilities inherent in the integration of the contemplative with the feminist; at the same time, she underscores for me the importance of resonant attachment central to both epistemological viewpoints. Her notion of the personal presents itself as one that can be used within feminist-contemplative writing pedagogy to denote presence. Specifically, Haraway supports an understanding of the person(al) *as* the "particular and specific embodiment" (1991c, p. 190) that makes meaning-making possible. As its etymology suggests, the personal in contemplative pedagogy is about the fleshy person, relating to one's body, which is understood within language but maintains presence beyond it as more than the simple object of our inquiry. By learning to accept our bodies as agentive and resistant to our attempts to overpower them with mental directives, yoga teaches us to approach ourselves as embodied and to be self-aware of the consequences of our materiality. Respect for and awareness of our materiality are equally important. A contemplative notion of the personal is therefore opposed to the expressivist notion of the personal as the psyche as well as the postmodern notion of the "personal" as an epiphenomenon or rhetorical construct, indicated by the offset quotations. The body, and so the personal, is always mediated by language but never overwritten by it.

Incorporating notions of the personal as embodied presence into composition pedagogy means accepting our students as "bodies who aspire to write" (Kazan, 2005, p. 392), or as writing yogis who use the skill of the embodied imagination to create a diverse body of knowledge that integrates the intelligence of the material. I use the term, "writing yogis," to press the similarities between the process of writing and yoga and to stress the usefulness in integrating these processes. I present the characteristic skill of writing yogis as the "embodied imagination" to forward a notion of how the writer becomes part of her text as she both writes herself into being by reflecting, reliving and rewriting her experience—we are written through language—*and* also finds lived reality and material meaning in the experiences that bring her to the act of composing—our bodies press language into shape.

Presence, or a materially-inclusive sense of situatedness, places us in the physical body as much as it situates us in discourse communities and social, ideological systems. The conception of resonant presence upon which contemplative writing rests thus refigures agency as a product of the harmonious interaction and co-constitution of the person and her environment—without losing the person to this environment through a diffusion into it. As such, contemplative writing is embedded in a figuration of agency as springing from our material attachments and the body's status as agentive in forming these. The knower-writer's material placement, her "specific and particular" body in relation to other bodies, guarantees her epistemic potential; without it, she could neither connect to others nor create meaning. This notion of embodied agency as stemming from a fullness of presence stands in stark contrast to standard performative definitions of agency wherein agency is seen as an extension of our social situatedness, disconnected from the material and completely discursive.

The movement toward integration here is harmonious with the practice of yoga, since the meditative moments of *asana* and *pranayama* teach the yogi to "transcend duality" and "to live with equanimity" (Iyengar, 2005, p. 16). Our attempts to understand the categories of writing-language and bodies-matter separately within our pedagogical practices tells us more about ourselves and our preference for "the politics of closure" instead of "differential positioning" than the nature of cultural construction or things themselves (1991c, p. 196). Closure is the opposite of presence, since presence necessitates openness to our environment, its changes and our dynamic position within it. Bodies become more than mere texts in contemplative approaches and material experiences literally matter even as they are also (re)written in the act of language expression. Corporeality is therefore neither "about fixed location in a reified body," challenging notions of authentic embodiment, but nor is it about "the body as anything but a blank page for social inscriptions" (1991c, pp. 195-197). Our fleshiness instead points to a material presence existing both within and beyond our linguistic representations and rules, primarily accessible to us via our linguistic mapping practices but also materially-situated and located within a larger world of matter to which we are accountable in the flesh. Understanding comes just as much from the body as the mind, since they are companionate composers in this epistemological picture. And because we can never experience the world from another's exact location, in another's body, the personal highlights a felt material integrity that even language cannot supersede, even if we can only make "sense" of this through language, and, through language, share our embodied experience with others. Contemplative writing pedagogies exchange words like "unique" and "authentic," which have previously tagged along with the personal, for words like "located," "mindful," "flexible" and "responsible." These are words that invite resonance and connection.

Once we view the personal as an expression of our bodies as well as our minds, we are dually required to rethink and expand our notions of situatedness. Because it views the body as more than a house for the mind or empty stage on which cultural scripts can be performed, the full (material-discursive) presence called for in contemplative writing differs from the more popular postmodern versions of social situatedness that constructivist writing pedagogies typically promote. No more can we simply refer to situatedness as a metaphor for socio-cultural placement; now we must also see it as about specific embodiment, about presence.

Butler's notion of the "constitutive outside" is an example of how situatedness and thus agency is typically construed through language, rather than through matter, and represents the limits of this view. Butler's construal is significant within composition studies since her theories of performativity, which rest on this notion, have been normalized within our disciplinary scholarship. Of the constitutive outside, Butler states,

> [t]here is an "outside" to what is constructed by discourse, but this is not an absolute "outside," an ontological thereness that exceeds or counters the boundaries of discourse; as a constitutive "outside" it is that which can only be thought—when it

can—in relation to that discourse, at and as its most tenuous borders. (1993, p. 8)

The constitutive outside carves out a space for excess within language by way of marking the unintelligible against the intelligible, bringing the other about. Importantly, this theorization allows Butler to argue for the social construction of gender while also questioning the inherent tie between sex and gender. The result, however, is that "[s]ex is resourced for its representation as gender, which 'we' can control" ("Haraway, 1991c, p. 198). To take this to writing itself, the writing body is resourced as subject, which teachers can similarly control.

While it may initially seem to be a liberating deconstruction, dismantling the biological category of sex (synecdoche for the writing body) forces the body to be the handmaiden of culture, or worse yet, an empty puppet waiting to be controlled by cultural, historical and semiotic forces. This view of language's total encapsulation of reality limits the potential *for* change and our potential *to* change as Fleckenstein remarks. For,

> [w]ithout bodies—those instances of flesh that disrupt the consistency of style and that point to a signification before and beyond language (Gallop 14-20)—no resistance of systemic transformation can be effected … nor can individuals cast themselves as agents of change because the uncertainty of deconstructed positioning erodes the embodiment necessary for agency. (Fleckenstein, 1999, pp. 284-285)

Agency and situatedness are recursively linked. We fundamentally change the notion of what it means to be agentive when we remove it from the body, and this change renders great losses. Fleckenstein urges us to refuse the disconnection of agency from the body by theorizing embodied writing as entailing both immersion and emergence, two techniques of situating ourselves. Immersion requires us to attend to the particularity of bodies, remembering that we experience our cultural placement materially, and emergence means we also accept the ways we are culturally constructed (1999, p. 297). Together, these orientations help us to construct a fuller conception of agency as it relates to contemplative writing practices.

Kazan illustrates how these paired acts of immersion and emergence can be mapped onto our classrooms. She claims the necessity of exploring how bodies *mean* in educational spaces like the writing classroom. If we think of immersion as "feeling out" bodies, we begin to see how this is pedagogical work we always do but rarely reflect upon as teachers. Kazan urges us to recognize these immersive practices and argues that as different bodies come together to comprise the corporeal text of the classroom, they begin to appropriate meaning in particular ways based on how their embodiments play off one another. The writing classroom is a situated space of learning because of the ways bodies are physically related to each other, meaning that bodies emerge in particular ways because of the social space of the classroom itself. For instance, the physical placement of the teacher at the front of her classroom materializes her authority and differentially positions her as removed from her students even if her body shares certain physical characteristics with those students, such as young age or popular dress (Kazan, 2005, pp. 380-381). Embodied writing pedagogy is always a mix of language and matter interacting together, meaning together. Contemplative writing pedagogy asks us to be mindful of this mix.

EMBODIED EMPIRICISM AND CONNECTION

Without attention to presence, it is easy to ignore our students' embodied differences. If we expect non-defensive openness from our students as they stretch their learning in our classrooms and begin to question the knowledge claims they import, we must meet them with a flexible mind and also a willingness to be changed by *their* inquiry. Contemplative knowledge by presence requires this flexibility in the face of change and within the presence of another. What the contemplative suspends, then, is the default move to see students' personal experiences as reducible to constructions able to be mapped onto cultural grids and chalked up to ideological saturation.

An example of how the refusal of the embodied and situated dimension of personal experience might work in a standard classroom guided by the tenants of social constructivist pedagogy is present in Karen Paley's analysis of Patricia Bizzell's writing classroom. Paley sits in on an undergraduate writing class dedicated to training peer tutors. While Paley remarks that the overall tone of the class was warm with "no evidence of confrontational pedagogy," she does conclude that Bizzell works to reframe students' comments so as to minimize the importance of personal attachments and maximize the cultural import. She states that Bizzell "welcomed personal commentary [from her students] only when it was explicitly linked to social, 'representative' issues" (2001, p. 187). This is evident in an example of the ways Bizzell validates students' readings of Patricia Williams' essay Crimes without Passion. Paley transcribes a students' response to Williams' essay and then Bizzell's response to the student during a classroom discussion:

> Sarah: I think there's a connection between all the stories that she tells, a lot of them have … the issues she's proposing, how

those issues came about as part of her development. So there's
a personal aspect of why she's so engaged in these issues.

Bizzell: I think this is a really important point, that she relates
her personal story and the issues; and Sarah's quite right that
one way of doing that is by developing it over time, showing
that it's something that has been an issue for her since she was
young. So the stories that she tells about herself are not just
personal stories, they are representative ... and I think that's
very important. (quoted in Paley, 2001, p. 185)

There is a "submerged disagreement" during this class that remains unnoticed and/ or unacknowledged by the teacher, according to Paley (2001, p. 185). As her quote indicates, Sarah thinks there is a connection between a person's individual "development" and his/her engagement with certain ideas and this likely is rooted in the ways Sarah experiences the impact of her material reality on her process of making meaning. Paley notes that the subtle disagreement between Bizzell and her student, Sarah, is indicative of the ways in which personal experience tends to be subsumed under the label of "socially representative" in order to stress how the self is a social construct and therefore not *personal* in the ways students like Sarah might articulate; it contains no material presence and can thusly be linguistically explained away through catergorization. As with Kazan's dance teacher, the method of instruction sanctions rather homogenous writing subjects, not writing bodies with difference.

Bizzell's treatment of the personal demonstrates the ways student experience becomes interchangeable when it is divorced from material agency and when students are not allowed to claim interiority through presence. It's in this context that Spigelman writes *Personally Speaking* as an attempt to allow students like Sarah a relative hold on their experiences while addressing a general anxiety over experience, displayed by Bizzell in Paley's study. But, as I indicated earlier, Spigelman's project purposely emphasizes "the *construct* that is personal experience" (2004, p. 60), and doesn't go far enough to reclaim the materiality of experience, and therein, embodied presence. This isn't Spigelman's aim anyway, as she is more interested in addressing the potential of personal writing to be a rhetorically-valid form of argument and not a mutt-breed of the writing classroom. But, it is mine. So while I do not take issue with Bizzell's attempt to teach her students the ways personal stories have cultural resonance, I do count as a pedagogical loss the implicit hierarchy between the social and the individual body as well as the flattening of all individual student bodies that her comments normalize.

Contemplative pedagogy dismantles this hierarchy; it focuses on the relationships between the personal and the cultural in ways that allow the person to stand *with* and not *for* the social by calling upon the critical power of his/her embodied experiences, refusing, as well, to ignore the embodied differences of varied bodies. Contemplative writing focuses on the process of knowledge-making as reflecting and analyzing a series of material experiences that reveal the complex construction of the individual as she takes shape in a cultural and social environment, but also as she marks that environment by means of her material embodiment and interconnectedness. It exchanges narratives of authenticity for those of situated positioning and humility. Engaging in contemplative writing practices means that we accept positioning as that which grounds knowledge claims and reclaims the body of the author. The personal is more than representative; it reveals the author's lived material investments and full corporeal presence. The classroom as well as the page should reflect this.

Haraway's notion of situated knowledge, or the material-discursive meanings we create from our experience, gives feminist contemplative writing pedagogies a means of articulating the importance of presence for embodied empiricism. Contemplative pedagogies forward a view of experience as much a material reality as a narrative construct. It is true that "'experience is not—indeed, cannot be—reproduced in speech or writing, and must instead be narrated'" (Brodkey, 1987, 26, as quoted in Spigelman, 2004, p. 11), but the process of shaping goes both ways, and so needs to include the ways our bodies and experiences beget our interpretations. I believe a feminist attitude of humility is best when approaching these issues in order to counter the tendency to mastery which often leaves us illogically claiming that our narration of experience somehow voids its materiality or that the sharing of emotion or agency disallows the intent of either (Amhed, 2004; Cooper, 2011). In order to realize fully contemplative writing, we need to see it as engaging in situated knowing and thus producing situated knowledge. If knowledge is always attached to the knower, we need to be wary of deeming the narration-reflection of experience a ventriloquizing act on students' or author's parts, one that is merely representative of the social. Indeed, the practice of material mapping is arguably a more responsible practice of viewing knowledge-making as it does not elide difference at the level of our bodies.

Situated knowledge is a feminist epistemology based on "particular and specific embodiment" (Haraway, 1991c, p. 190) which produces "partial, locatable, critical knowledge sustaining the possibility of webs of connection" (Haraway, 1991c, p. 191). These webs privilege attachment through "passionate construction" and "resonance, not ... dichotomy" (Haraway, 1991c, pp. 194-195). Based on these definitions, we can first see how situated knowledge highlights the ways materiality and discursivity are tangled in our webs of meaning, making it impossible and particularly senseless to separate them. Nor does it behoove us to overwrite matter as a function of the social insofar as it is reduced to nothing more. Situated knowledge consequently places the writing yogi in the center of the meaning-making process and refuses to ignore how her body is implicated in her knowing as materially placed and connected to her experiences. These experiences spatialize the writer in the world, literally positioning her in definite yet dynamic ways. And, "[s]ince yoga means integration, bringing together, it follows that bringing body and mind together, bringing nature and the seer together, is yoga" (Iyengar, 2002, p. 48). Situated knowing is itself therefore an enactment of yoga.

Put differently, situated knowing within contemplative pedagogy is an epistemological practice that changes our understanding of *how* we come to know by locating knowing within individual, writing bodies not a transcendent realm of truth or a social "body" motored by language. Because experience is a product of this mutual, interdependent composition, and not just linguistic, writers "do not simply 'reinterpret' [their] experiences through a new discourse; experience also enables reinterpretation … experiences are discursive, but they come, at least in part, from somewhere else, not 'just' from discourse in an endless devolution" (Hirschmann, 2004, p. 327). We accept the idea that experience can be understood entirely through discourse when we read it exclusively as a text. Taking on a contemplative viewpoint means we acknowledge that there is more to material reality than discourse and that a position of openness which validates our ultimate lack of mastery over a material world to which we belong but can in no way ever comprehensively view is a strength not a limitation. Contemplatively, language cannot fully capture our embodied realities even if we use it to explore our place in the world: "[t]hat such experience can only be shared *through* language is important to recognize. Indeed it may be a crucial dimension of the standpoint notion of shared experience that we communicate about it through language, but discourse cannot exhaust the 'reality' of experience" (Hirschmann, 2004, p. 327).

In other words, situated knowledge requires writers to exhibit mindfulness of themselves, others and their environments. When engaged in building situated knowledges, we are exercising mindfulness by contextualizing what we or others are experiencing within how and why we are experiencing it. That situated knowledge engages us in a practice of mindful knowing has a second implication: situated knowledge is metacognitive, asking us to be reflective of our thinking and to monitor it by investigating: 1) what we are experiencing; and 2) how we are experiencing it. This metacognitive process of investigating our thinking about what we know and how we got to those knowledge claims is at the heart of contemplative mindfulness. In their operational definition of mindfulness, Bishop et al. agree that mindfulness is itself a metacognitive process and can be used to develop the practitioner's reflective skills: "the notion of mindfulness as a metacognitive process is implicit in the operational definition that we are proposing since its evocation would require both control of cognitive processes (i.e., attention self-regulation) and monitoring the stream of consciousness" (Bishop et al., n.d., 11). The following interchapter will take up these ideas and will explore this link between mindfulness and metacognition in greater detail. But, at present, it is important to recognize how metacognition through mindfulness necessarily entails acceptance of an interiority of thinking that invites acceptance of a writer's "center" in line with contemplative theory.

In sum, situated knowledge can be used to develop contemplative writing pedagogies to make them not only more theoretically sound but also more pedagogically generative when enacted in the classroom. This kind of knowledge rejects traditional modes of detachment and seeks to relate the material and discursive at the level of meaning and enact it at the level of our bodies. "To a yogi, the body is a laboratory for life, a field of experimentation and perpetual research" (Iyengar, 2005, p. 22). Situated knowledge is consequently what gets made on the page and in the classroom when we engage in contemplative writing and teaching practices.

Contemplatively, embodiment is a necessary condition of meaning making, fixing the body as the origin of knowledge. Its inseverable connection to the body is what makes this knowledge "partial" as well as "locatable." *What* we know accordingly changes too. If the process of knowing is primarily experiential, we must entertain seriously our personal experiences and work to interpret them critically without losing their embodied reality. In this feminist epistemology, "[d]iscourse and reality are in close relationship, but they are, nevertheless, distinct" (Hirschmann, 2004, p. 327). Indeed, we can understand the relationship between discourse and material reality as one of companionate composing. Understanding can come from *interpreting* an experience not just *having* it so that we can connect to each other even when we experience our embodiments and material-discursive worlds differently (Hirschmann, 2004, p. 329). In short, we can situate ourselves within the context of an experience through our imaginative interpretation of it without having experienced the actual context ourselves; the meeting of discourse and matter is a generative one that enforces the companionate relations between the two.

As such, situated knowledge is an interested practice of knowing through connection, partly because we use language to communicate with others and partly because we are always connected to others through our shared materiality. The commonality of our materiality, which can be seen as a dynamic common ground even if it is experienced or embodied differently, gives situated knowledge a relational, "webbed" orientation that establishes it as a method of connected knowing. Connected knowing values the historical, social and experiential and is characterized by its stance of openness, a continuous deferral of closure, and by the recognition of our need to join with others (Belenky et al., 1973, pp. 113-123). It understands difference through connection, not distance. In contrast to separate knowers who experience the self as autonomous, connected knowers experience the self as always in relation in "webs of connection." This is what Hart may mean when he argues that contemplative pedagogy is founded on a "more *intimate* and integral empiricism that includes in the consideration of the question a *reflection on ourselves* and on the question itself" (Hart, 2008, p. 237, emphasis added).

Intimacy easily gives way to loving care. The worldview of interrelatedness required by situated knowledge entails "the loving care people might take to learn how to see faithfully from another's point of view" (Haraway, 1991c, p. 190). The position of interrelatedness and attachment to other matter—people as well as other objects—is what makes this knowledge responsible where responsibility is seen to stem from a understanding both of the interest of all knowledge claims as well as the perspectival limits of personal, experiential knowledge. This notion of connected responsibility as giving weight to knowledge claims contrasts with the distance from the self other methods of knowing suggest. Here, one can be critical *and* personal *and* present at the same time since it is impossible to rise above the self. And neither does this connection to the knower invalidate the public use value of her knowledge claims: as stated above, the map cannot exist without the map maker, but it can be read and followed by others.

Situated knowledge is therefore not the same as subjective knowledge. It recognizes multiple standpoints and not just one. It is interested in a dialogue between the personal and the social that doesn't collapse the integrity or importance of either. Situated knowledge accommodates a multiplicity of embodied standpoints since "differences in experiences produce differences in standpoints" (Hirschmann, 2004, p. 320). Recognizing difference is part of the contemplative knowing process for, "if knowledge is developed through experience rather than an abstract world of 'Truth,' then different experiences will yield different bodies of knowledge" (Hirschmann, 2004, p. 320) which can be strengthened by being placed in relation to each other—bodies mean in relation to other bodies even if they retain individual integrity. So even though lived moments are accessed through the social filters of language and cultural histories, the stories we develop to explain and capture these moments are always threaded to the moments themselves and the "having" of the experience. Certainly "the stories we tell ourselves of our experiences come filtered through the collective subjectivities of our social and cultural relationships, so that our interpretations of experience are not simply individual" (Spigelman, 2004, p. 63) or personal, but they are also not simply social or textual—interpretations of material realities presuppose those lived realities without exhausting them. These material acknowledgements fly in the face of our pedagogical tendency, following from cultural studies theory, to discredit our students' ordinary experiences as naïve or interchangeable. Experiences of the student (and teacher) instead need to be both validated and analyzed.

Outside the dance studio, Fleckenstein in her recent book, *Embodied Literacies*, similarly points out the way we neutralize student bodies in academic discourse and the resistance this promotes. In this book devoted to increasing the scope of literacy to include the embodied nature of imagery, Fleckenstein argues that teaching academic writing is not just about developing a successful psychological identification to a middle-class life and value system, as represented by Bartholomae's discussions of appropriation, but is also about adopting a physiological identification since the act of writing "imposes on students the bodies of white, heterosexual, middle-class males," (2003, p. 49) an argument well-made by feminists from Virginia Woolf to Helene Cixous and Jane Tompkins. The stakes are much higher than discursive reconstruction. Fleckenstein's analysis is meant to give us a greater understanding of student resistance, but it also highlights how our narrow application of social situatedness tends to hide these embodied consequences of learning to write.

To authorize student experiences, we must explore how they come from a body self-reflexively affirmed and differentially positioned. This will be the subject of my next interchapter. Because our bodies as sites of knowing are embedded in culture and language, our experiences are not self-evident but they are where we must necessarily start. To ignore them is to "pretend to disengagement" (Haraway, 1991c, p. 196). To work toward engaged analysis, the situated knower is the first to examine how her experiences are not solely her own, and how she must accept her partiality and join with others through language; nonetheless, situated knowing does not reduce materiality to discourse since our materiality can actually function as a challenge to discourse (Hirschmann, 2004, p. 325) since it is agentive. As a result, situated knowledge presents a third space of rhetoric-cum-referentiality.[14]

If we use situated knowledge as a guide, we begin to see the ways we can discuss personal stories and experiences that reveal writers' attachments while allowing them the material integrity they deserve. To promote critical thinking, we can teach writers to look for and analyze the incongruences that arise in these stories because writers are situated in ways they cannot fully recognize due to their embodiments, their specific placement and presence in the world. Students can begin to see dissonance as a result of not only competing worldviews but also different configurations of felt materiality. I explore in the next chapter the ways we can discuss how the writer is materially, culturally and ideologically situated and how we might approach these dynamics of being a body in the world simultaneously as strengths of writing and knowing and also signs of our need to join with others. I show how in strong contemplative writing, authors tend to recognize the partiality of their knowledge claims even as they validate them as a product of their experiences and feelings.

Teaching students to think critically about their embodied experiences typically presents a challenge. In contemplative writing pedagogies, this is a challenge that can be met at both the material and discursive levels through the lens of situated knowledge. Situated knowledge can be used to develop embodied pedagogies of writing to make them not only more theoretically sound but also more pedagogically generative when enacted in the classroom. Situated knowledge as an epistemology becomes a way to rethink our current writing approaches; situated knowing as the connected practice of generating meaning can help us to work toward changed writing practices—ones that recognize fully students' agentive embodiment as writers and the material weight of their experiences. As it rejects traditional modes of detachment, relates the material and discursive at the level of meaning, and enacts it at the level of our personal bodies, situated knowledge is what gets made on the page and in the classroom when we engage in contemplative writing and teaching practices.

The process of metacognitive reflection within feminist contemplative writing pedagogy also maintains connections between thinking and feeling. Writing yogis, who are situated, connected knowers, integrate personal knowledge with knowledge from others and weave together reason and emotion, using the insertion of the self in knowledge production as a way to generate reflection and analysis, a process I will show the workings of in the next interchapter. As a result of the complexity of this localized process of making knowledge, writing yogis who employ connected knowing with mindfulness have a high tolerance for openness and ambiguity (Belenky et al., 1973, p. 137). This is why situated knowers are after "resonance" and not hierarchy. Viewing situated knowledge through the lens of connected knowing allows us to see how it is both a process of situated knowing as well as situated feeling. This means we must begin to recognize the critical power of our feelings as they are a part of the knowledge we create. I will turn to the ways contemplative writing suggests the futility of divorcing situated thinking and feeling in Chapter Three.

INTERCHAPTER TWO: HABITS OF YOGA MINDS AND WRITING BODIES

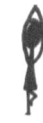

> Your practice is your laboratory
> —B. K. S. Iyengar

> Yoga helps my writing more than anything else I've ever done.
> —Student

In the contemplative tradition of yoga, it is customary for yogis to set *sankalpas,* or intentions. Intentions are reminders that yoga is just as often practiced off the mat as on it; that daily living is as in need of mindful purpose as *asana,* or posture practice, is. Intentions have always been a key part of my yoga practice and have more recently become just as important to my writing process.

Lately, I've been working with the intention of noticing without jumping to judgment—of simply being present and aware of the moment. I set this intention because in the last few months, I've been rushing through my practice and have ended my time on the mat with vague feelings of frustration. Putting my intention to work, I was able to see what's causing this habit: my struggles with forward folds. Just as I folded over my legs during sun salutations, I felt frustration bubble up and the urge to move quickly into the next pose. Staying with this feeling, I came into contact with self-judgment for not being as flexible as I'd wish to be. Knowing why I am disappointed won't necessarily stop this feeling, but that's not the point.

Now when the automatic lick of disappointment arises, I follow through with my intention to allow these feelings to surface. But rather than ruminating on what I can't do just yet, I purposely refocus on the sensations of my body, so that I maintain full presence in that moment of my practice. To learn from it. Can I notice the space in my back body? Is my weight in my heels? Am I lengthening my spine before I fold forward? Am I linking my outbreaths to my downward movement?

This intention-driven learning will eventually lead me to the flexibility I desire because it will increase understanding and acceptance of my present reality. And while respecting my current limits, it will also encourage me to set goals for what I wish to work toward. These are lessons I transfer to my writing. I apply this present-centered attention to my writing process so that when I encounter stuck spots of writer's block, I rush toward awareness instead of ruminative judgment, which can discourage me from writing my way through these spots or understanding why a restful break may be necessary.

As with all contemplative traditions, contemplative education forwards the intention of awareness. Contemplative writing pedagogies are built on mindfulness in much the same way my yoga practice is. That is, they teach writers how to develop a practice of mindfulness and how to pay attention. These are skills all learning requires but few of us teach explicitly in our writing classes. We assume students know how to be aware, but that they often choose not to be. Attention is a switch that some aren't willing to flip. This refusal leads to shoddy drafts written in one sitting the night before a paper is due. I've found that this understanding of attention isn't quite right; my students often don't know how to sustain attention over the extended periods of time they may need to write and revise a paper or read and reflect upon a lengthy academic text. This is why they wait until the last minute, which brings at least a focusing urgency if not the attentive awareness of a carefully-carved reflective space. The multitasking methods of students' everyday lives have them toggling between Facebook, the latest writing assignment, their cellphone (vibrating to alert them to a new text message), the television on behind them and the Pop-Tart® in front of them—all at the same time. The continual practice of splitting attention creates a habit they understandably find hard to break. So while my students complain about the consequences of such split focus for their writing and learning, they tend not to know *how* to choose another method or *what* other methods exist. Indeed, they feel they have no choice at all.

Even when students do limit distractions enough to classify themselves as "paying attention," they tend to approach this process statically, as psychologist Ellen Langer notes in A Mindful Education. Langer reports that when high school students are asked what it means when a teacher tells them to "pay attention," either to "(a) keep your eyes steady on it or (b) think about it in new ways," almost all students think the instruction means to "keep the stimulus constant" (1993, p. 48). No wonder students find this hard to do; it's the complete opposite of multitasking, which requires moving, albeit erratic, engagement. What's more, when most writing teachers ask students to pay attention, I'd wager we're after more than simply having students keep an idea still and fixed in their minds. When I invite my students to "pay attention" in class, for example, I want an active engagement that questions and creates paths for insight and creativity. It is this latter, more fluid and flexible form of attention that contemplative writing pedagogies teach students. In contrast to paying attention as a means of fixing something in your mind, these pedagogies ask students to develop a practice of noticing: thinking actively about an idea or concept and seeing it from multiple perspectives without automatically rushing to judgment. Contemplative pedagogies do this by linking awareness to context and to the body, which interacts dynamically with the world.

When writers learn contemplative practices like yoga and meditation, they develop a felt understanding of awareness that changes the *intention* of paying attention and teaches them that attention is a choice under their control. For instance, when students attend to their breath during *pranayama*, or the practice of breath control, they develop a moving awareness that follows their inbreaths and outbreaths; they do the same when they learn to link inbreaths and outbreaths with *asanas,* or postures. In my application of contemplative pedagogy to the writing classroom, I ask students to integrate the mindful practices of yoga *within* their writing processes, seeing them as continuous with the typed or written words-on-a-page they inscribe. Not only does this teach students that mindfulness is developed by bridging body and brain, cultivated empirically and situated in their own flesh, but it also develops their conscious awareness of meaning as material, of writing as physical. Mindfulness is a kind of full body training, then, that helps writers develop flexible attention to thoughts, ideas and themselves as dynamically situated in material environments. In other words, contemplative writing pedagogies explicitly teach students *how* to pay attention. And, when students exhibit increasing flexibility of attention through mindfulness, breaking from automatic response and moving toward embodied, reflective awareness, they have earned their contemplative moniker, "writing yogis," discussed in Chapter One.

A flexible mind isn't only valued by contemplative educators; it has also been deemed one of the necessary eight "habits of mind" integral for college writing success by the recently-released Framework for Success in Postsecondary Writing. This report represents a joint effort of both secondary and postsecondary educators to examine what skills, attitudes, behaviors and experiences all students need in order to assume a level of "college readiness" (2011, p. 1) prior to their pursuit of higher education and to determine what they'll need in order to exhibit learning excellence once enrolled in college writing programs. In short, this document marks a guiding intention for our field. As writing instructors, we should intend to develop students' habits of the following: curiosity; openness; engagement; creativity; persistence; responsibility; flexibility; and metacognition. As with contemplative practices, these habits of mind are practical and help students make choices about their learning and literacy.

103

In addition to knowing rhetorical skills and how to apply them, the Framework establishes these skills as necessary for encouraging students to take an active role in their educations and for fostering the kinds of critical-creative thinking that will help them excel not only as writers but also as college-level learners and literate citizens. Habits of mind are tools for developing awareness. By prioritizing habits over discrete skills, even if these have a place too, this document argues against formulaic or rigidly standardized writing curricula; the habits are necessarily learned through activities and assignments that engage students in writing for real-world audiences with genuine and not solely assessment-related goals in mind. While rhetorical skills are necessary, the authoring agencies of the report suggest that they cannot be successfully developed and deployed by students who are not simultaneously encouraged to cultivate certain methods of approaching the learning and writing processes. In these ways, we might see the Framework as underscoring the importance of developed writerly awareness, or of approaching writing mindfully. Ways of thinking about writing become just as important as the means of actually doing writing.

When I first read the Framework, I was struck by the congruity between the goals outlined in it and the reflective remarks my students made in their writing blogs about what they learned by integrating yoga within their writing processes and how they embraced mindfulness as a writing intention, concept and tool. Looking at both what writing teachers say we want—at least as represented within this recent document—and what my students say they have learned in the reflective writings recorded on their blogs, I would like to outline in the following pages how contemplative pedagogies can help sustain and foster the habits set forth in the Framework, goals we as a field have established as intentions for our instructional practice. By looking to the situated knowledge students produce within their blogs, I will argue that contemplative pedagogies provide us a novel and useful means of enacting these intentions with mindfulness and give our students means and methods of attending to their somatic development as writers.

The advantages of putting a well-researched, field document that represents the collective wisdom of composition studies in dialogue with my own and my students' experience of using yoga to rethink the writing process are many, but the one I have been most interested in within these pages is how new pedagogies can help us reach the goals of post-secondary writing instruction while encouraging us to examine the means we use to accomplish the educational ends we say we desire. I want to suggest that not only does a contemplative approach to the writing process help students develop the habits forwarded by the Framework, but also that it uses means that develop them as habits of mind *and* body, penetrating students' lives at a deeper level and offering them a foundation to approach their educations contemplatively and their writing mindfully. These two words are never used directly in the Framework, but they still penetrate its implicit call for an education that cultivates inner awareness and teaches students to live more attentively in the world, which they can do to a greater degree when they are in the habit of seeing themselves holistically as body-heart-minds.

As I've earlier explored, feminist contemplative pedagogy is a thoughtful, embodied pedagogy responsible to our flesh and maintained by theories and practices that honor the intelligence of the body. Contemplative pedagogy recognizes the link between awareness and self-reflection and values how the body and mind must work together to synchronize acts of knowledge creation. Feminism adds a richer understanding of the stakes of respecting organic bodies as sources of intelligence; it refuses the split between body and mind complicit in so many of our pedagogies and traces this split back to fundamental structures embedded within Western patriarchy. It's been my intention throughout this project to show how feminism adds a valuable dynamic to contemplative pedagogy by making contemplative practitioners aware of how transformative a heuristic and practice of mindfulness is for the writing classroom.

Mindfulness, as both a heuristic for contemplative pedagogy and a body-minded habit achieved through consistent involvement in contemplative practice, can be seen as a frame for the eight habits of mind listed in the Framework. Consequently, development of these habits results from engaging students in the feminist contemplative writing pedagogy I've been utilizing, one that incorporates yoga within the process of writing. Other contemplative exercises may be used to cultivate a similar transformational mindfulness, as I noted in my introduction. And, certainly as Rick Repetti argues, "[a]lmost any classroom exercise may be transformed into a contemplative one simply … by slowing down the activity long enough to behold—to facilitate deep attention to and intimate familiarity with—the object of study, whether it is a slide, textual passage, equation, claim, or argument" (2010, p. 14). While there are just as many ways of enacting contemplative pedagogy as any other pedagogical approach, the use of yoga to engage students contemplatively has been my focus in this project.

While I could go into great detail about how each of these eight habits of mind are developed and strengthened by bringing yoga into the writing classroom, I'd like to focus on three that I believe to be especially illustrative: openness, persistence, and metacognition. The Framework defines *openness* as a "willingness to consider new ways of being and thinking in the world," or a responsiveness to differing and alternate perspectives, using these to inform our own; *persistence* as "the ability to sustain interest in and attention to short- and long-term projects," or the ability to follow-though with tasks by applying focus and developing attentiveness; and *metacognition* as "the ability to reflect on one's own thinking as well as on the individual and cultural processes and systems used to structure knowledge," or the ability to examine the writing process and how it structures knowledge and the contextual merits of personal and/or substantiated evidence (2011, p. 5). As defined, these three habits can be understood to largely encapsulate the others. Many would agree that anyone open to the learning process would have to maintain a strong sense of curiosity and eagerness to explore new and unfamiliar ideas, for instance. I will use these three representative habits to examine students' responses to contemplative pedagogy and the ways yoga can support a writing process that strives for mindfulness and, therein, rhetorical awareness. As students use yoga to navigate their writing processes, they generate habits of mind that both ensure their present-moment success (since they are approaching it purposefully) and enable them to transfer theses habits to other endeavors as their whole beings become engaged in learning.

HABITS OF THINKING AND BEING: OPENNESS

At the beginning of every semester, I revisit worries about the risks I take as a young faculty member engaging in pedagogy that attempts to teach writing in novel ways, ways some may deem strange because of their unfamiliarity. But the professoriate worries me much less than the student body. The bulk of my fear stems from the risks I take in the classroom, in front of students who I always imagine to be less interested in alternative ways of knowing than they turn out to be. Rather than allow these fears to mindlessly rule my teaching choices, however, I pursue them with the same mindfulness I advance in my application of contemplative pedagogy and practice as a yogi. These fears teach me that the value of taking risks as a teacher is that I might model for students what a contemplative process of learning looks like. They also remind me of what Ellen Langer claims is key to a mindful education, the "process of stepping back from both perceived problems and perceived solutions to view situations as novel" (1997, p. 110). Through Langer, I recognize that my understanding of appropriate pedagogical action in my writing class is shaped by what was modeled to me as a student and by the accounts of successful teaching I studied as part of my graduate education. Both the lore and the theory I inherited. But when I see each class as a novel way to explore what writing feels like to me as a writer and where my own mindful explorations of the creative process have led me, I allow openness to dictate my teaching and not only tradition.

Similarly, perhaps the most obvious benefit to an integrated practice of yoga and writing in the classroom is how it establishes a learning atmosphere of openness to various ways of thinking and being in the world at large, beyond that with which students may feel the most comfortable, because it is habituated and known. My self-coined "yoga for writers" practices—or other contemplative practices for that matter—are not standard fare in first-year writing classes at my university. Introducing my writing students to yoga is so different, in fact, that my first challenge lies in helping them piece it into the larger learning puzzle that college presents. While students enrolled in my courses are encouraged to open up the ways they think about writing and practice it, none of their friends or roommates are going through the same experiences in their composition classes, marking my classes and my students.

Despite the challenges that novelty brings, I have continued to use these practices and have taken even more steps to more fully integrate yoga and writing in my classes—utilizing a practice of *pranayama* to start our sessions as I outline in the next interchapter, for instance. I have not simply charged onward as a pedagogue committed to contemplative writing who has found an integrated approach to yoga and writing theoretically-fulfilling: yoga has indeed become a means of literally embodying the writing process and teaching students to think of themselves more holistically than is typically encouraged in secularized school settings. This thrills me as a contemplative practitioner and a feminist teacher. Yet, as much as I love theory, my classrooms recursively inform the theoretical side of my pedagogy just as much as the reverse is true. I've continued to mark myself and my classes in these ways because I have found this integrated approach so meaningful to students that they practice yoga everywhere they write, even in between the library stacks—close to the cubbies in the library at which they type their drafts on laptops—defying normative social codes and risking embarrassment for the sake of a better writing process. I've simply never had students take so many learning risks nor reap so much understanding about the writing process before. If my students are willing to do yoga in the library, I am committed to keeping this pedagogical practice available to them.

My students' appreciation of contemplative writing practice takes time, however; their openness to a new writing experience is limited by the immediate academic demands ("Will this get me an A?") and social pressures they face ("Will this make me look stupid?"). Because I respect their concerns and want them to know I do, I pointedly tell students of our intentions from the very first day of class. I explain that I am interested in what changes when we think of the writing process as making both physical and mental demands on us and how we might construct a writing life[15] that connects the writing process to our persons as wholes and not just our need to fill pages for assignments. I talk to them about how yoga is being used in K-12 classes and teacher-training programs.[16] I also discuss with them the ways mindfulness-based stress reduction (MBSR)[17] has proven to help students learn better and feel less stressed by the incredibly high demands of college life and academics. These are issues they relate to because they've been forewarned of these demands and begin to feel them from the moment they begin their college careers. Even so, I invite students to come talk to me about their reservations and/ or excitement and ask them to bring me questions or concerns immediately. While our practices are optional, I tell them I'm going to encourage them to try yoga, to take a risk with the hopes that it will pay off big for their growth as writers. By the end of the semester, most will have participated and will agree that it was a worthwhile risk. Taking risks is an essential element of developing an open-minded approach to learning.

Before we do yoga together, a process I narrate in my preface and conclusion, my students and I talk about it a lot and connect it to a larger discussion about writing as a physical process of creating meaning. This gives us a reason to investigate writing as a topic onto itself in our classroom, keeping us grounded in that even as we may explore additional themes within our units. Thinking about the writing process as physically-demanding is new for students, as I explore in my first interchapter. As I detail there, we work through what writing has meant to us, how we've approached the process, and how we've often ignored our physical writing habits. We begin to pay more attention to those. Do we listen to music when we write? Should we? What are the benefits of sitting up straight or writing in lounge chairs? What changes when writing at desk chairs or while lying on beds? How do our physical locations impact what we write about or how we write? These are all questions my students first grapple with as they learn to pay attention to their writing bodies.

Using their physical writing habits as a bridge, I explain to students that our yoga practice will be a common language for us to have conversations about the physicality of writing and the ways we create meaning through experience. Some students remain a bit apprehensive about using yoga to help develop their skills as writers, even if they are catching on to the idea of contemplative writing and beginning to think of themselves as writing bodies—a first step in developing the flexibility of a writing yogi. Jimmy represented this common reaction of surprise in a blog post. Explaining that he discussed our planned but yet untested use of yoga for writing with friends, Jimmy notes that it is "a little unusual that we would do yoga in an English class, and everyone I told was like, 'Yoga in English? What?'" The incredulity represented here is usually a result of students' ignorance about contemplative practices and their general uneasiness to do anything that seems "weird" or out of the ordinary. Important to his testimony is Jimmy's record of sharing our upcoming yoga practice with friends outside the course. Because there isn't much in the way of a contemplative educational community outside the bounds of our class at my university, Jimmy's peers have no way of understanding our mission and only Jimmy, for whom the process is new and untested, can explain. For Jimmy, in particular, this was a major concern because he was an incredibly social male who often repeated his desire to pledge a fraternity on campus as soon as he was able. With difference sometimes seen as deviance, Jimmy was likely concerned that our practices would mark him in undesirable ways and provide him experiences to which his peers would not be able to easily relate.

The other reaction I most commonly receive is excitement, although not necessarily for the yoga practice itself. In many cases, my students are excited for a break from the standard, college class routine. The fact that we won't be having a traditional class and will be doing something out of the ordinary is thrilling to students who hear and see classmates and teachers go through the same motions day after day. Sharing in this spirit, Jimmy's classmate, Tori, remarks, "No matter what, at least we get a break from sitting in the classroom." It's the same thrill of change that motivates another student response: "My first day of class I was told that we were going to be doing yoga to help us with the writing process. 'YOGA?!' I thought. I guess so, why not try something new? After all, college is about new experiences and adventures." Because this craving for something completely novel isn't captured by our normal classroom activities, it can create new excitement for learning and passion for writing.

Aside from benign skepticism or interest in a new adventure, every semester there are a handful of students who have practiced yoga on their own and are committed to our integration of yoga and writing because of their appreciation of contemplative practice. These students, who often self-describe as athletes, often note how their bodies crave movement, even or especially when learning: "I always move my legs when writing. I have a hard time learning, listening to anything if I'm not moving. I learned to read while spinning in a circle. It just helps me," says Gwen. This craving for movement characterized Gwen, for as long as I knew her, as she was always coming or going to an intermural practice on campus. Gwen even dabbled in yoga before entering in my class because prior athletic coaches encouraged the practice and cited its many benefits for athletes. I've found this last group of students to be the minority, even if they are also the fastest-growing segment in my classes. Every semester I see more students who've voluntarily practiced yoga, sometimes inside and often outside of the classroom, prior to their experiences in my course. These students help to sway some of the more resistant simply by their positive presence and willingness to bring these two worlds together.

Despite initial apprehension, many students develop an embodied understanding of yoga after practicing it. For instance, Jimmy, who was reluctant at first because of fears of being criticized by friends, notes that after our first practice of yoga,

> explaining [to inquiring friends] the reasons why we did yoga actually opened my eyes to the connection my professor was trying to make between the body, mind, and writing. Yoga required physical flexibility and strength .... Writing is somewhat the same way .... One can't get frustrated with how their first draft ends or how there are errors throughout the writing process.

Jimmy's comment mirrors research that learning new skills is best prompted by the adoption of a learning mindset geared toward openness and not closed, ruminative judgment. Openness can minimize the negative effect of stress, enhance feelings of calm and regulate negative emotions like frustration (Roeser & Peck, 2009, p. 129; Holzel et al., 2011, pp. 542-544). Jimmy has a felt understanding of this link between yoga and writing after just one practice. His comments testify to what happens when writers practice mindfulness, which yoga forwards as attention that suspends immediate judgment: they remain calm in the face of "error" and become more open to progressive development. Openness also provides writers the mental and physical support Jimmy's classmate, the very active Gwen, details in her reflection: "[Yoga] does fit in with the rest of the classes so far. Yoga is about being in the moment, which is what you have to do when you write. If your body is loose but awake, your mind will be too .... Yoga can help us write because it helps us focus our mind and body on the task at hand and be open to actually doing it." Being open to the body's intelligence and recognizing its impact on their attentiveness are common themes among these student reactions.

Students like Jimmy and Gwen, when read closely, can point us to the ways a "yoga for writers" practice encourages writers to listen to their bodies and to see them as sources of learning and meaning. In other words, my students are beginning to recognize how their bodies are implicated in the processes of knowledge production; they are beginning to see meaning-making in terms of situated knowledge, as explained in Chapter Two, as their bodies are placed centrally in the process of knowing and implicated in their thinking about thinking. As writers start listening, they learn a practice of being open to themselves, of approaching their intelligent bodies with wonder. In other words, students learn a process of self-monitoring, which can be used to better process new information. Mountain pose or *Tadasana* (see Figure 2), the first standing pose my yoga teacher, Holly, and I teach students as part of our first "yoga for writers" practice, facilitates the development of such self-monitoring. To practice this pose, students stand up straight with their shoulder blades pressed into the back and widened in order to sink them down and create space in the back-body.

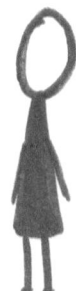 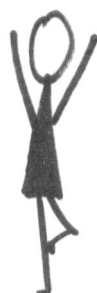

Figure 2. *Tadasana* and *Vrksasana*

This pose always amazes students because it is as simple as standing up straight, but in ways that make them aware of how engaging such an ordinary action can be when done with awareness of the body. When they concentrate on their bodies in this *asana* and begin to monitor their movements, students discover that they shift their weight between their feet and sway with the action of standing, something they've often not noticed before. When students subsequently learn tree pose, *Vrksasana* (see Figure 2), an advanced balancing posture that requires them to further direct to these subtle movements, Holly encourages them to accept sway as a constant in yoga practice, movement that must be met. I remind them that the same is true in writing, for without attention to movement, we cannot learn which side we favor, potentially impairing our balance if left unchecked. These corrective actions are less about dominance over the body, which could lead to injury, and more about working *with* the body, understanding it in order to make adjustments that entail a union of flesh and brain.

In their article on the advantages of adopting contemplative educational practices in traditional learning settings, Robert Roeser and Stephen Peck argue that practices like yoga cultivate conscious awareness of the self within an ethical-relational context because they engage students in these kinds of situated adjustments. That enhanced self-monitoring leads to students' awareness of how both their bodies and brains are involved in processes of creating meaning is reflected in Ann's response: "Tree pose ... [is] my favorite. It's my favorite because for some reason I can balance pretty well in it and it represents balance in your life, which I'm working on ... personally ... and in my writing." And, as she practices tree pose and others like it, Ann's ability as a writer to stabilize new information in memory and develop subject matter knowledge while connecting this new information with prior learning improves because of the ways her brain changes during her practice of mindfulness through movement (Baime, 2011, p. 47). From developing her working memory to opening up her perceptions of writing, Ann changes her identity as a writer and the stakes she places on her process because she uses yoga to navigate the physical and mental demands of writing.

Ann's response also strikes a hopeful note. Her intention of balance testifies to the ways yoga helps develop not only students' openness to writing but also their receptivity to themselves. In other words, Ann is learning to exercise self-compassion. Compassion applied to the self and others is a goal shared by all mindfulness practices. In their article, Roeser and Peck note that the compassion taught through contemplative practice creates better students because contemplative learners "take a kind, non-judgmental, and understanding attitude toward [themselves] in instances of pain or difficulty rather than being self-critical" (Roeser & Peck, 2009, p. 129). Essentially, mindfulness training "facilitates an emergence of a compassionate awareness and a change in the emphasis of the experienced sense of self" (Tirch, 2010, p. 119). Given that so many of my students describe the writing process as painful and that we often use dissonance to talk about learning, such an attitude is essential in our composition classrooms. As Ann balances in tree pose, she cultivates mindful awareness of how the body sways despite her best attempts to stay perfectly balanced. She learns that there is no such thing as perfect balance and that balancing is a matter of moving with the sway of her body and not staying rigidly still, which is impossible. This teaches her that stability isn't a fixed quality and that she must be plastic in her approach to strength.

As Ann does, all students can translate this plasticity to the writing process as a lesson in working with their bodies rather than overpowering them. From there, it is a short leap to also accept the fluctuations of the world and our environments in our writing habits so that incorporating "sway" as opposed to rigidly sticking to one idea to the utter exclusion of other points of view is not a sign of failure. The embodied lessons of balancing poses like *Tadasana* or *Vrksasana* serve as living metaphors for how yoga practice can serve writers, reminding my students to approach their and other bodies with openness, listening to all sides before hastily making a movement in their writing. The poses also serve an immediate, material function for students, opening them to the intelligence of their writing bodies.

HABITS OF MIND AND BODY: PERSISTENCE AND SUSTAINED INTEREST

Persistence, as defined by the Framework, entails commitment and attention. It requires students to try on new ways of thinking about the writing process and new methods of managing their composing sessions and to follow through with these tasks over the course of the semester. The first lesson of persistence students learn when using yoga for their writing is that they must frequently practice both processes together for noticeable gains. After completing our first "yoga for writers" practice, blogs requesting their initial responses (some of which I share above) and subsequent class discussions, students begin using *asana* in their daily writing sessions. (See my appendix for a sample handout given to students outlining poses and connecting them to the writing process). We also start our practice of in-class *pranayama* and meditation, which I detail in my next interchapter. It is important that students practice this integration during class time and that they also approach themselves as writing yogis outside of class, for it is during these times that they execute a great deal of their composing.

Since I ask students to complete a weekly writing blog, wherein they document their process for our class (and, if they desire, for other classes as well), I also request students use this blog as a space to keep themselves accountable to incorporating yoga into their routines, before, during and after their writing sessions. Again, it is important that students see our yoga practices not as deviations from our class work but rather as connected. When students opt out of our yoga practice, I give them the option of using some other sustained physical practice like running or regular walking to take its place. Allowing students the autonomy of choice is a lesson in responsibility and also gives them nothing to react or rebel against, since our practice remains a suggestion rather than an inflexible requirement. Perhaps because of this flexibility, most of my students do choose to use yoga; I've only ever had a small handful of students who used another physical practice in place of it. And, even those students still typically joined in for our classroom-based yoga, even if they infrequently practiced on their own.

If most continue to practice yoga willingly, all typically rise to the challenge of thinking about the movement of their bodies as an integral part of the composing process. And they benefit. Zach is a student who stands out because of his motivation. A type "A" myself, I recognize this quality in my students almost instantly. He was one of those students who brought all the course texts to class on the first day "just in case" he'd need them. Zach's organization and question-asking secured his success in my class but was driven by his perfectionism, which caused him a great deal of undue stress. Zach was won over by our practice of yoga because he found great relief from writing frustration in his practice—and therein a greater commitment to the growth of his papers. He states, "When I'm stuck, I can stop to breathe or [to do a] pose instead of staring desperately at the computer screen. Through the break I can relax and write longer and better without the added frustration." Zach is successful as a writer because he exchanges desperation over the long-term nature of the writing process with short-term productivity guaranteed by yoga "breaks." These breaks, he claims, become a part of the writing process because they help him reengage his attention rather than disengaging it, so much so that he believes the break and his process are continuous: "In fact, it is not so much a 'break' as it is part of the physical writing process. I can honestly say yoga has helped me develop as a writer." Part of the way yoga has "helped" Zach is by developing his persistence, entailing the kind of commitment to an ongoing writing task that my student here demonstrates. The sustenance Zach finds in his yoga-writing practice is well-supported: research completed at the University of Kentucky found that students who engaged in contemplative practices like meditation when taking a break from their studies showed enhanced brain functioning superior to those who napped, watched television or talked with friends (Grace, 2011, p. 113).

Commitment can also be attributed to student writers' abilities to trust that persistence will pay off in the end. Contemplative acts build that trust as they increase the strength of executive control processes. Students who engage in them are more likely to appreciate delayed gratification (Roeser & Peck, 2009, p. 129), such as the benefits of rewriting a paper many times, which may reap rewards including more confidence in writing abilities and a higher grade. These delayed rewards begin to seem more attractive rather than the instant gratification of procrastination. Research has shown that with continued focus on contemplative awareness this self-regulatory "capacity to inhibit the dominant response tendency is associated with both social-emotional (e.g., better stress management) and academic (e.g., higher SAT scores) benefits" (Roeser & Peck, 2009, p. 129). Take Sasha, a gifted artist, as a case in point.

Sasha claims that while she always knew procrastination wasn't what you were "supposed" to do, there was previously something practical about waiting for the surge of energy she got when writing a paper at the last minute; even if it was confused and disorganized, the paper would get done. Plus, procrastination provides more time for her to "do the other stuff [she] enjoy[s]." But developing a corporeal orientation to the writing process with yoga shifts her understanding of the effectiveness of this method so that a paper "done well" begins to mean more than simply "done." Instead of being quickly written the night before, she notes that a recent paper for our class "took many different writing and brainstorming sessions to complete as well as two conferences and peer review." For this student, becoming a writing yogi means slowing down and listening to her writing body—an impulse opposite from her typical tendency to procrastinate, which places unreasonable demands on her body and mind. Overriding her habitual responses by listening to her body not only makes the writing process more enjoyable, less stressful and therefore more accessible on a day-to-day basis, but it also helps my student write more imaginatively and carefully, factors that will make her drafts more persuasive which could (and did) lead to earning higher grades.[18] Extending the amount of time she works to draft her essays also increases her ability to entertain new ideas as her drafts grow and incorporate her peers' ideas and challenges to her thinking brought on by conferences, as her remarks indicate. This impulse of mindfulness, of slowing down and paying attention, is characteristic of a pedagogy that fosters contemplative awareness.

My students not only exhibit newfound persistence when completing their writing projects, but they also demonstrate corresponding changes to their thinking about writing. Noting his personal goals in using yoga for writing, Kevin states in a blog that growing in his abilities as a writer is equally important to committing himself to the idea that such growth takes time. Slow persistence is a remarkable insight for this particular student, a highly motivated second-language learner who desired a native speaker's fluency from the moment he entered my class as a first-semester international student. Yoga gives Kevin a new model for progressive growth:

> All I need to do to get better at a particular pose or my flexibility in general is that I need to at least try my best. My pose will be the closest to the one that instructor demonstrated in my best ability. I think it is same in writing. There always will be better writers than me or anyone in the classroom. There will be the best example on particular writing style or the way to write well in general. I am not saying it is impossible for anyone to get that level, but it will be pretty darn difficult. However, if I try my best … I can say that is a great achievement.

Kevin recognizes that persistent effort, trying his "best," may not make his writing process perfect or help him flawlessly execute yoga poses but that perfection need not always be the goal. Rather than encouraging students to be dismissive of their efforts, learning limits helps students set realistic goals that keep them motivated to write and learn.

When students like Kevin see writing in terms of yoga, they keep in mind how they must notice gradual improvement in writing as in *asanas* and that flexibility—of body and mind—is hard won and slow to develop. Such acceptance may be attributable to the ways that contemplative practices like yoga have been shown to help students develop "motivational mindsets" (Roeser & Peck, 2009, p. 129) that give them both concepts and scripts to use when navigating their abilities and any setbacks to their goals. That is, because "contemplative practices require the mastery of challenging mental and physical skills (e.g. sitting silently and watching the in-coming and out-going breath or maintaining a particular physical pose) (Roeser & Peck, 2009, p. 129). It follows that "engagement in these practices ... provides numerous ways of understanding oneself and one's attempts to learn and be resilient during the process of learning" (Roeser & Peck, 2009, p. 129).

Native speaker, Abby, who shared Kevin's introspective nature, certainly expands her self-understanding by engaging in yoga, and this appreciably benefits her writing. She states that with yoga, she is able better recognize when her body and mind need more time to grapple with difficult ideas. Abby notes that yoga teaches her to slow down since always pushing herself to her limits leaves her burned out and ready to quit:

> When writing does not go well, I will stop and do some yoga to relax my body and mind, rather than forc[ing] myself to go forward. Not only does yoga make the body feel more focused, it relaxes the mind more than anything I've ever done outside of running .... [Yoga also promotes] self reflection which helps me put things in perspective and can yield clarity and bring the body and mind closer .... I feel that the most important thing that yoga shows us is that slowing things down and having alone time can really clear the mind and body.

If the Framework suggests that persistence is about learning to "follow through, over time, to complete tasks, processes, or projects" and "grapple with challenging ideas, texts, processes or projects" (2011, p. 5), both Kevin's and Abby's testimonies reiterate the ways healthy persistence can be supported by engaging students in contemplative writing processes. Yoga, in particular, teaches them that persistence is sustained by learning how to best keep the fires of energy burning long and slow over a period of time. Indeed, their comments exhibit persistence with a contemplative edge of self-compassion. Putting things "into perspective" is both a means of treating oneself compassionately and of placing a writer's perspective in the body.

Studies on the merits of contemplative education show that students who develop self-compassion are more likely to approach setbacks with a positive mindset and less likely to correlate academic failures with their sense of self-worth. Self-compassion is specifically linked to students' understanding of moment-to-moment fluctuations in perception. And, monitoring of these fluctuations is taught by balancing poses, as detailed above. With my students in mind, we can see how yoga helps writers develop an increasing acuity becoming aware of habitual responses. Learning to redirect these automatic responses can play a key role in fostering informed and self-endorsed behavioral regulation, which has long been associated with well-being enhancement (Brown & Ryan, 2003, p. 823). Self-compassion inspires greater feelings of confidence and competence among student writers and an increased, intrinsic desire for growth and improvement. Students who exhibit self-compassion are more likely to focus on their learning and improvement as opposed to their performance in comparison to others—key for the transfer of learning.

In contemplative pedagogy, compassion is developed by tuning into the body, which strengthens the areas of the brain that stimulate caregiving behavior (Tirch, 2010, p. 118). "Being aware of my body helped during the writing process because when I felt tired and sore from working and writing, I knew to take a break," says Sasha, echoing Zach's earlier comments. Because Sasha spent a great deal of time drawing (her favorite pastime), she notes that she also used these moments of learned awareness to monitor her art sessions as well. Even though Zach's worries stemmed from his ability to produce a successful paper and Sasha's from concerns for her waning creativity and tired body, both students benefitted deeply from yoga. Breaks, instead of becoming a waste of time, become a necessary part *of* rather than deviation *from* the writing process when my students attend to their writing bodies. And breaks embody the compassion these writers are learning to feel for themselves. Neither recognition is trivial. Sasha continues, "[i]f I try and overpower my body and complete too much in one session, I end up with poorly written paper that looks like it was written in a hurry. I am also a lot less creative when my mind and body are tired and need a break." With such attention comes a healthy dose of respect for how the body shapes the results of our writing sessions and our writing products themselves.

Mindfulness doesn't just encourage focused attention on the experience of writing at any given moment; it also helps writers find peace within themselves when they feel weary or worn out. Whether we practice mindful breathing as we move through yoga poses or as we sit quietly and solely focused on our breath, "[o]ur resentments, angers, regrets, desires, envies, frustrations, and feelings of superiority and inadequacy" fall away …. Of course they return, but the remembered experience of peace acts as proof that these obstacles are not insurmountable; they can be detached and disposed of (Iyengar, 2005, p. 97). And when they are disposed of, we can refocus on our goals. Yoga teaches students that embodying their imaginings of focus and peace helps them to reenter them. Holly and I stress to students the importance of remembering the peace and balance they create during practice; for, if they can remember this, they will be assured that place is never too far away. But, if they can't recapture this peace, they can just as easily re-create it. This is why another student, weary and about to completely lose focus, practices yoga in the library, where she happens to be writing her paper:

> I was working a long period of time with no breaks on an assortment of assignments, not because I was in a rush just because I had the time. I studied to the point that I couldn't concentrate and my body just felt like I needed to walk around. Since it was a crammed library day I did not want to lose my spot and I was still leery of leaving my stuff around, I went in an aisle of books and started doing [*asanas*].

That my student is willing to risk being seen doing yoga in the stacks loudly speaks of her belief in its efficacy for her ability to sustain focus. The need for her mid-library practice can be summed up by one of her classmates' responses: "The yoga rituals bring in a focused, calming energy that allows me to expand upon and spread out my writing. I find I can actually write for longer periods of time if I incorporate different exercises throughout the writing process." With such comments, my students demonstrate that they are learning how a united and calm body and mind are necessary for awareness and that yoga can aid them in cultivating such calm attentiveness.

Because yoga helps students develop mindfulness, it can increase the quality of their attention, which has a direct impact on their success as writers. Just ask my students. Their experiences with a yoga-writing practice show that "the practice of focusing awareness on a single object (e.g. a physical pose, the breath) promotes sensory inhibition and a 'relaxation response' … and can cultivate nondirective, open, vigilant, and receptive forms of awareness" (Roeser & Peck,

2009, p. 128). My students respond to these gains because they often combat debilitating stress and mental anguish over the writing process that interferes with their ability to focus on the task at hand. Practices that enhance their mindfulness develop "a greater ability or willingness to allow and be present with negative emotions rather than attempt to suppress or avoid them" (Robins, Keng, Ekblad, & Brantley, 2010, p. 119).

HABITS OF MIND AND BODY: METACOGNITION

The data I continue to collect from my classes convinces me that approaching writing through yoga has the ability to increase writers' embodied awareness of themselves and the world in which they live because it places their writing bodies at the center of the composing process and not at the periphery. In turn, student writers become more attentive to the other bodies to which they are connected by virtue of their shared materiality, prompting both self- and other-awareness. In other words, yoga helps students develop a corporeal orientation to themselves, to others and to the writing process by making them mindful of the ways their bodies help create meaning in their papers. They see how their bodies shape their perspectives as well as the evidence they cite to support their arguments, and they notice the physical dynamics and demands of the writing process itself. In the contemplative tradition, mindfulness is used to describe awareness of the present moment and attentiveness to experience. Rather than getting ruminatively "caught up with the 'internal chattering' of the mind or other contents of awareness, individuals who engage in mindfulness practice learn to observe their thoughts, emotions, and sensations in an objective and receptive manner, focusing on the *process* of awareness, rather than the *content*" (Robins et al., 2010, p. 118). Developing mindfulness allows writers to become aware of and then monitor their thoughts and feelings. With awareness, they can begin to regulate their thoughts and emotions in productive ways that transcend automatic habits and thoughtless reactions. Practices like yoga that cultivate mindfulness are not simply relaxation techniques then, but are "rather a form of mental training to reduce cognitive vulnerability to reactive modes of mind that might otherwise heighten stress and emotional distress" (Bishop et al., n.d., p. 6). For instance, restorative poses such as *Savasana*, a supine position on the floor, encourage us to become aware of our feelings of restlessness, imbalance or rigidity so that we may release and relax into an attentive calm we might not otherwise achieve if we never consciously attended to those feelings.

Because mindfulness engages students in monitoring their thoughts and redirecting them, it can be understood as a metacognitive skill, or one that engages students in thinking about thinking (Bishop et al., n.d., p. 11). The Framework for Success in Postsecondary Writing defines metacognitive abilities as including the ability to analyze epistemology, or the ability to reflect on one's own thinking in ways that puts it in dialogue with "cultural processes and systems used to structure knowledge" (2011, p. 5). In writing courses, metacognitive acts draw students into an analysis about their thinking processes and about their writing practices and the ways writing creates meaning (and doesn't simply reflect it). This analysis encourages writers to make epistemological conclusions about context, place, form and audience—or, most simply, the situatedness of meaning. Attentiveness to situatedness is a direct application of our yoga practice and is embodied every time students make choices about which poses to integrate from our yoga labs. I encourage my students to apply the embodied knowledge they gain from the integration of yoga and writing strategically and mindfully based on their needs, developing physical writing habits that are best for them: those who find a practice of restorative yoga poses helpful to promote focus and clarity are encouraged to use these; others who find more energetic poses beneficial to generate ideas are encouraged to use those. And all are encouraged to mix and combine these methods since their bodies and minds are dynamic and therefore unification of their energies can proceed in different ways on different days.

Because they are both involved in generating new knowledge about the visceral and situated nature of writing and in contextually applying these ideas to their own composing processes, students who practice yoga and writing together are, I argue, thinking metacognitively on a consistent basis. Using their blogs to spur their reflections simply enforces this kind of thinking; writing about writing leads to thinking about thinking. What's more, because students approach such metacognition from an activity of mindfulness, they more readily assume a learning orientation "characterized by curiosity, openness and acceptance," the state of a mindful mind (Bishop et al., n.d., p. 9). The return on this orientation is open acceptance of writing bodies, as I've shown, and a growing acceptance of the physicality of the composing process. Students' blog responses further enact what we might understand to be the three primary elements of metacognitive thinking: planning an approach to a given learning task, monitoring comprehension and evaluating progress toward the completion of a task (Lv & Chen, 2010, p. 136).

Approaching Writing

As I've illustrated in my previous sections, consciousness of how the body bears on the process of making meaning changes how students think about and complete writing tasks; students confront the ways they may have narrowly categorized the writing process as a "brain activity," a conception that previously encouraged mindlessness in regards to bodily influences on their writing. Now conscious of their writing bodies, they begin to attend to the shaping powers of materiality on meaning and on the meaning making processes of writing. For instance, Terry notes that a regular practice of doing yoga helps him "get ideas for writing." Terry believes that if not for yoga, his brainstorming would suffer:

> Had I forced myself to sit and write in front of a laptop, I doubt if I would come up with ideas so easily. Had I limited myself only to the mental aspect of writing, I would never have enjoyed writing at all. Who would love writing if he has to sit for three straight hours and struggle to write his papers? This is the reason I become obsessed with writing overnight.

Terry examines the mindset he takes into the writing process and finds that yoga helps sustain motivation because it gives his body a release from the stress of staring at a blank Word document. His reflective response represents the ways he has learned to use yoga specifically for brainstorming, which has worked so well that he has become "obsessed" with the writing process as a result of our class. If metacognition entails being able to notice changes to ways of thinking and to adapt execution of the writing process in order to respect these new ways of thinking, then my student here demonstrates this ability.

Students also begin to do the metacognitive work of unpacking how their bodies' intelligence transfigures the meaning, and not just the transmission of ideas, in their writing. Terry tells us how he begins to tap into the intelligence of his body in order to create more effective and creative writing sessions. In contrast to his yoga-writing practice, approaching writing as only a mental task, as he did prior to our course, is a "limitation," he tells us. The metacognitive act of thinking about writing spurred on by our yoga practice and supported by our classroom discussions helped another student reconceptualize writing similarly. Peter states that he began "to see writing as an animating physical task rather than a monotonous mental chore." He reports in a blog post that this changes his relationship to writing, as he begins to understand how the process of writing was physically demanding in ways he hadn't typically respected, as all-nighters meant to finish papers ignored up until their due dates confirmed. New understandings of the writing process, of "writing physically" as he calls it, also breed new ideas about meaning creation for this student. Reassessing the content of his writing, Peter remarks that even when he isn't writing in first person, his ideas "originate from what we see, what we hear, what we smell, what we taste, what we feel, with everything being alive and activated." Conceiving of writing in this way brings my student not simply motivation for process drafting but also increased respect for the ways knowledge is sensory and visceral.

Monitoring Comprehension

While I've already explained the ways contemplative activities such as yoga help students develop a self-monitoring mindset to the end of increasing their attention in my section on persistence, this mindset also applies to the metacognitive processing that these activities encourage. As they explore their changing approaches to the writing process, students must come to terms with how changes in the execution of the writing process positively impact their understanding of writing too. As they write differently, their concept of composing substantially shifts.

Sarah's new appreciation for writing as an embodied process is such a liberating one for her that she begins to critique standard forms of academic writing. She sees these in a new light because of how successful integration of yoga and writing is for her. While she frames her understandings in common language since I provided little framework and no jargon for these insights in class, she specifically questions the masculinist bias inherent in those standards of keeping "yourself out of your writing, even when it's you always writing." Instead, she believes it's important to "respect our bodies" as writers. Writing a decidedly feminist statement in regards to the liberatory potential of embodied writing, Sarah claims a newfound appreciation for the importance of experience as evidence in her writing and how "remember[ing] how our bodies affect our emotions" can help her draft more persuasive arguments. While these new recognitions specifically "help when writing more creative pieces," they also pique her interest in hybrid, critical arguments that require recounting and analyzing personal experiences alongside other forms of substantiated evidence. These inclusions are "something that we don't usually do, we usually compartmentalize our minds from our bodies and even parts of our body from our body as a whole" according to Sarah. Developing her feminist message, she goes on to say, "and this happens more with women; women tend to be partialized." In a conference with me, Sarah disclosed why she was so passionate about critiquing the ways women are encouraged to see their bodies in parts: this stemmed from her experience with seeing fellow competitive figure-skaters succumb to disordered eating because of the pressures they felt to stay thin. Sarah noted that she herself had only just begun to value her strength as a competitive athlete over her thinness. Because Sarah thinks "it's harder for women to think of their bodies and minds as wholes instead of individual parts," she believes in the feminist potential for contemplative writing practices that validate the body's felt intelligence. For Sarah, a female writer and a lifelong figure-skater, the embodied imagination of the writing yogi is necessarily a part of a feminist epistemology which changes her understanding of how certain choices in writing lead to the creation of different ways of knowing and being in the world. Certainly, these are life-changing conclusions that were spurred on by our contemplative agenda.

Other students note changes in their understanding of writing on a smaller scale, in terms of their confessed weaknesses. A weakness many students' metacognitive remarks coalesce around is the value of focus and the means to sustain attention, which is helpfully developed by our practice of yoga. Summarizing her peers, Samantha states, "My personal writing pain comes in the form of focus." But yoga helps Samantha to relax: "I was trying to brainstorm over the weekend and I laid [sic] on the floor and put my legs up and thought. My roommate thought I was crazy, but I think I actually like what I thought up. I was relaxed and when relaxed, it's easier to connect to my body and mind .... Hopefully my narrative will benefit from this connection and ease I felt while brainstorming." And it does, perhaps because she develops this metacognitive insight: "When writing [the second paper] I kind of answered each point individually, and I think next time I'm going to try and avoid doing that. Instead I'll try to make [my analysis] more focused and connected so I'm not just answering one part and then another." From this metacognitive vantage point yoga becomes a means of problem-solving. Devon uses yoga to solve his problem of jumpiness as well: "Yoga gave me a way to see inside my writing. My writing can be extremely jumpy from time to time. Yoga paired with the breathing exercises helped minimize the jumpiness ... with my improved focus, my papers began to make more sense and stick to one topic."

That yoga can help my students "see inside" their writing and can help them describe the process of creating drafts that exhibit cohesion and clarity testifies to the power of contemplative acts to bring about metacognitive awareness of the writing process. Yoga gives writers new methods to plan the writing process and work through the stages of writing from drafting to revising. It also helps them monitor their understanding of audience, exhibiting a sense of mindfulness about how audience, purpose and organization are connected.

Self-evaluation

Finally, yoga writing can give students a new method for self-evaluation, or for gauging their learning progress and determining successful completion of writing goals. My student Sarah says, for example, "The whole process [of using yoga for writing] has also brought me to see writing on a grander scale," because yoga exercises "allowed for self-evaluation" when writing. Yoga helps Sarah become a more flexible thinker and writer. And as she notes, "I think that emotionally, I got a lot more relaxed about writing, and that is growth." Sarah continues her self-evaluative reflection and states that yoga helped her see how writing should be like "a person on a page, and that's not perfect." What this means to her is that rather than hiding from ambiguity in her writing, she should embrace it:

> Confusion can be shown in the paper, though not by confusing the reader, and instead by asking questions about the world and our being ... though initially chaos may ensue from the lack of concrete knowledge, the ultimate result of imagination and exploration of self will be incredible ....
> Then we can continuously redefine ourselves without fear of change, without fear of loss.

While Sarah's formulation may be one of the more direct and perceptive I've received, her classmates responses rally around the shared understanding that by alleviating anxiety and prompting self-evaluation, yoga helps student writers successfully cope with ambiguity at the level of meaning making in their writing. That yoga becomes for students a new way of understanding writing as well as a set of practical tools to help them cope with these negative emotions of writing is telling of the lessons students can potentially learn as writing yogis, which have both imaginative as well as lived consequences.

Sarah is not alone in her growth. Nicole also believes that yoga helps her to stop ruminating on her "flaws" as a writer and helps her to accept them as points for future growth, not signs of present failure: "To be able to know that you can improve in the future [as a writer], and to be able to find your own flaws is growth. I don't understand how I was never able to do that before." And this growth helps Nicole approach writing more joyfully, now that she better recognizes her own thinking: "My writing process is so much more relaxed, so much less tearful, when there is less pressure on me to make it perfect, and I never really realized until this year that the majority of that pressure was not placed upon me by my teacher or peers, but instead by myself." This revelation transforms my student's attitude toward writing and learning and releases the intense pressure she felt when writing previously—so much so that she confided in me shortly after writing this blog that for the first time, she enjoyed writing and hoped to find more ways of making it a part of the fabric of her life.

As my students have shown, contemplative writing pedagogies can help writers develop habits of mind consistent with the Framework for Success in Postsecondary Writing. When I began this chapter, I noted that I would not fully explore the cultivation of each of the eight habits the Framework lists out of a concern for space but would instead focus on just three. In the exploration of those three, I believe it becomes clear how one habit unfolds to reveal the others. Before I end, however, I'd like to draw everything together by reviewing this unfolding and bringing these three habits in dialogue with the others once more. I remain general in my closing, hoping the reader will reference specific examples from my case studies above.

Because approaching the composing process through yoga necessarily involves students in a novel process of inquiry that has them asking creative questions about the physicality of the writing and meaning-making process, it piques students' *curiosity* about how writing works, what it can do and also about different, culturally-contingent ways of knowing. In thinking about how their bodies shape the writing process and, therein, the written product, students confront the Western conception of knowledge as removed from the body and complicate this with Eastern concepts of the body-mind exemplified by our practice of yoga. This *engagement* helps them *open* up to new ways of thinking and being in the world, especially those that are less dualistic. As students notice how simple things like posture affect the meaning they create in their papers, they begin to wonder how knowledge is impacted by even larger material and social factors, so much so that one of my students developed his own theory of situated composing he later reduced to a personal mantra of "where I write is what I write." This is *creativity* at its strongest.

Understanding knowledge as situated helps students *flexibly* adapt to context, genre and audience and to recognize the value in certain writing conventions, which can help foster communication with and through a myriad of differences. Practically, students also learn to work with their own embodied differences as writers, figuring out how and when to integrate yoga poses and techniques in their writing process in order to become more *persistent*, focused writers who can sustain interest and attention. Sustained interest, students learn, is partly accomplished by learning to be *responsible* to both their writing bodies and minds, which cannot be easily accomplished in all-nighters that produce a first-and-last draft paper. From a yogic perspective, these lessons of navigating our inner worlds translate to external applications so that as students become responsible to their own bodies, they extend this responsibility to other material beings by virtue of their connectedness to them. In the writing classroom, this application starts with students' classmates. Students come to see how peer review, for instance, derives its meaning from its ability to foster resonant, material connections between writing bodies with dissimilar ideas, less so because of its function as a tool to catch errors before a paper is due.

All these efforts represent a new way of thinking about the writing process as well as a new method of doing writing that includes attention to the body and a working with it. These changes, therein, encourage students to entertain a level of *metacognition* about their writing that may otherwise be absent or at least not enthusiastically exercised in classrooms where the reflective stakes are lower, often because students can mindlessly pass through while remaining within their learning comfort zones. My experiences have shown me how contemplative writing pedagogies encourage authors to reflect on themselves as embodied, as writing yogis, to experience the writing process as physically demanding and to recognize the writing product as materially saturated. With these habits of mind and body cultivated and enacted, students exposed to this pedagogy become embodied imaginers in all the ways I describe in previous chapters. In the next chapter and interchapter pair, I turn to the last element of imagining: feeling. Chapter Three explores how contemplative pedagogues might attend to feeling using understandings of flexibility from yoga and Interchapter Three tests these theories out, applying them to examine the consequences of integrating exercise of pranayama, or focused breathing, in the writing classroom.

CHAPTER THREE: SITUATING FEELINGS IN CONTEMPLATIVE WRITING PEDAGOGY

> It is difficult to speak of bodily knowledge in words. It is much easier to experience it, to discover what it feels like
> —BKS Iyengar, *Light on Life*

In 2003, UCLA's Higher Education Research Institute (HERI) began a multi-year study to document the emotional and spiritual development of undergraduate college students. Researchers based the study on the premise that institutions of higher learning "have increasingly come to neglect the student's 'inner' development—the sphere of values and beliefs, emotional maturity, self-understanding, and spirituality" (2005, p. 5). In 2005, HERI released its report on this study. This report found that of college students "more than two-thirds (69%) consider it 'essential' or 'very important' that college enhance their self-understanding, and a similar proportion (67%) rate highly the role they want college to play in developing their personal values" (2005, p. 6). Another 63% of students want college to provide for their emotional development (HERI, 2005, p. 6). These high percentages should give us pause. Our current educational default is to divide a student's so-called personal life and growth, what the study refers to as "inner development," from the critical enterprise we often take as the sole ground on which we can and should teach. But, this is not what our students claim they need.

The results from the HERI study directly support the pragmatic mission of contemplative education to teach the whole persons in our classrooms, taking an integrative approach to students' outer *and* inner lives—in precisely the ways they are asking that we attend to them. To learn in their bodies, students must consciously approach their thinking, feeling and being as joined. A contemplative approach is fueled by mindfulness, awareness cultivated by present-centered attention that seeks to watch and not immediately judge unfolding experiences, ideas and feelings, anything that passes through the filter of our mind-bodies. In their attempt to create an operational definition of mindfulness through a careful review of existing literature in both Buddhist and secular traditions, Scott R.

Bishop and his team of researchers note that mindfulness establishes a change in perspective when attending to our inner experience. That is, while open to present-moment experience when engaged in a practice of mindfulness, we learn to focus on the process of our awareness as opposed to simply its content. We become more process-directed. So, "in a state of mindfulness, thoughts and feelings are observed as events in the mind, without over-identifying with them, and without reacting to them in an automatic, habitual pattern of reactivity" (Bishop et al., n.d., pp. 8-9). Through this process of self-observation, we learn to monitor and regulate both our thoughts and emotions using a conscious mode of acceptance. This mode of acceptance is contemplative, not conventional; it does not reduce the self to its thoughts and emotions because mindfulness creates a space between perception and response. This space invites recognition not unconscious attachment, which can be used in a complementary process of delayed assessment and, perhaps, eventual change. These mindful self-observations are "meta" moments of awareness. Educators call this process "metacognition," naming the strategy that learners use to manage and monitor the learning process; contemplative practitioners, like yogis, call it "insight" for the same reasons. Because "mindfulness is thought to enable one to respond to situations more reflectively (as opposed to reflexively)" (Bishop, 1997, p. 9), we can understand it as a conscious strategy of metacognition.

Contemplative pedagogies that use mindfulness as a heuristic, practice and tool to build students' awareness therefore have the ability to increase students' development of metacognitive insight, as I explored in my second interchapter by looking at this term through the lens of the Framework for Success in Postsecondary Writing. This process has implications for the HERI findings: the cultivation of mindfulness through contemplative practice has the potential to increase students' self-understanding and, in turn, provide them with the tools to better understand their cognitions, feelings and personal values, characteristics of education that students claim to be missing in traditional educational structures. These structures, according to Fleckenstein, in privileging only the mind's role in learning, have "divided human beings from the affective or spiritual basis of learning" (1997, p. 26). Contemplative education's mission of mindfulness attends to students' whole being, addressing previous omissions of emotion and spirituality in learning. And because mindfulness involves both a process of rooting into oneself as well as shifting out toward others, as I've explained in earlier chapters, it can help students learn to pair inner awareness with social responsibility. Indeed, the integrative approach of the contemplative insists that we stop dividing our educational missions along an inner/ outer binary: it isn't possible to teach social responsibility without attending to inner awareness. In the words of contemplative educator Zajonc, "[w]e attend, the world forms around us ... and so on cyclically. In this way, attentiveness works back on us as formation" (2010, p. 91). Our students' emotional lives are intertwined, then, with their intellectual and civic pursuits.

Feminist theorist Allison Jaggar argued for an inclusive view of emotion years ago, well before Antonio Damasio (cf. *The Feeling of What Happens*) reasoned that thinking and feeling aren't divisible since the mind is embodied. Jaggar warned us that

> time spent in analyzing emotions and uncovering their sources should be viewed, therefore, neither as irrelevant to theoretical investigation nor even as a prerequisite for it; it is not a kind of clearing of the emotional decks, "dealing with" our emotions so that they not influence our thinking. Instead, we must recognize that our efforts to reeducate our emotions are necessary to our political activity. Critical reflection on emotions is not a self-indulgent substitute for political analysis and political action. It is itself a kind of political theory and political practice, indispensible for an adequate social theory and social transformation. (164)

Our pedagogies are nothing if not political, making Jaggar's statements valid for the contemporary writing classroom. In what follows then, I hope to examine the theoretical and the practical consequences of making emotions pedagogically visible in the contemplative writing classroom by teaching our students the skill of embodied imagining. Feminist theory within and outside our disciplinary bounds creates an exigency for such visibility within contemplative writing pedagogy and anchors my investigation of how we might enable students to become passionate, embodied imaginers, constructively engaging their emotions instead of simply managing or dismissing them. Such efforts support our students' quest for a meaningful education, as represented in the HERI findings.

In a spirit of inclusivity, I refuse the closure of defining feelings as entirely linguistic *or* organic and of delineating between cultural affect, psychological emotions or physiological feelings in what follows. Instead, I borrow education theorist Meghan Boler's comprehensive definition of feeling[19] as "in part sensational, or physiological: consisting of the actual feeling—increased heartbeat, adrenaline, etc." and "also 'cognitive' or 'conceptual': shaped by our beliefs and perceptions (1999, p. xix). If feeling is material, it also discursively shaped too: "[t]here is, as well, a powerful linguistic dimension to our emotional awareness, attributions of meanings, and interpretations" (1999, p. xix). A holistic definition of feeling appeals to me because it recognizes the organic body's shaping of emotion as well as the ways our feelings are always situated within a culture and a specific material placement in the world, a double gesture maintained by contemplative pedagogy and by yoga.

I will extend my previous analysis of Haraway's concept of situated knowledge, which I engaged as part of a contemplative epistemology in the last chapter, to include a corollary dimension of what I call "situated feeling" in the pages that follow. By recognizing how emotions and knowledge are entangled, I argue that feminist contemplative writing pedagogies give us ways of recognizing exactly how emotions impact writing and provide us a method by which they can be productively theorized and engaged within composition studies. As I locate my enactment of contemplative education within the practices and philosophies of yoga, I will suggest how we can involve our students in a situated process of feeling by teaching them an Eastern-inspired "emotional flexibility" that establishes feeling as part of the body's agency and reclaims it as a *teachable* skill with social effects. In simple terms, I argue that we must teach students, understood to be writing yogis in contemplative pedagogy, to approach their feelings with openness and resilience in order to become more flexible writers. But first, I briefly turn to the tendency to manage emotions, an impulse driven not only by our canons of scholarship but also by the teaching lore of our field. My discussion of emotion will, in the end, lead me back to the embodied imagination as a space wherein students' emergent body identities can be made agentive and the negotiation between situated thinking and situated feeling can become a means of meaning making and self-determination within the praxis of feminist contemplative writing pedagogy.

"FEELING LORE:" THE "PROBLEM" OF EMOTION IN THE PRACTICE OF TEACHING

Aligning criticality with thinking and consciousness with discourse has often had the unfortunate effect of maintaining the displacement of affect from the process of learning to write. Early critics of emotion in composition leveraged their social models against cognitivism, which, they claimed, ignored the impacts of language for the biology of emoting. Even so, while early cognitivist investigations of emotion have fallen out of favor for social-constructivist views of emotion as situated, Alice Brand's original message from those investigations that "[o]ur students need to be familiar with both the emotional and intellectual cues they experience that tell them they are ready to write, ready to stop, and ready to do a number of things in between" is as true and valid as ever (1985/1986, p. 11). The terms we use to explore these cues have changed, and compositionists such as Laura Micchie, Susan McLeod and Lynn Worsham have asked us to re-examine early dismissals of emotion by critical pedagogues who did not find appeals to biology compelling. These women have attempted to reconcile early biology-based conceptions of affect with newer theories of discursive construction and social conditioning. Their scholarship has helpfully created a new wave of attention to emotion within composition studies, but it has often done so at the cost of entertaining the body as an agentive emoter, a feature of contemplative writing pedagogies. This is a point I will develop in the next section. For now, I'd like to focus on what should trouble us all: even with a surge of new scholarship on the discipline and maintenance of our affective lives, the traditionalist contrast between reason and emotion continues to resonate in our teaching practices and the lore surrounding our discipline. If lore reflects a physical enactment of our theories, our teaching literally embodies the dismissal of emotion, and, with it, the writing body from our classrooms—no matter if we approach these from the lens of discourse or biology.

If we understand lore to account not only for the dissemination of knowledge in our field, but also the production of it, as Patricia Harkin calling upon Stephen North does (1991, p. 125), the persistent denigration of emotion as reason's inferior (female) mate is extremely concerning. If our rituals and practices of teaching writing do not account for the emotional experience of writing, learning and meaning-making, we do ourselves and our students a great disservice and justify the suppression of the body in composition studies. "Bringing lore to light" (Harkin, 1991, p. 138) can show us what works in the classroom and give needed merit to the embodied labor of teaching, but it also exposes the fault lines between our practice and developing theory. In this case, how recent efforts to theorize constructive models of engaging students' and teachers' emotions as part of the work validated and valued in the writing classroom have not yet revolutionized these classrooms—classrooms that in reality may be producing knowledge counter to those recent, progressive theories of affect. I argued in the last chapter that our situated knowledge, informed by our experiences, can be used as a means of making critical the integration of personal, embodied evidence and social analysis in the writing classroom. Here, I contend that the lore regarding the validity of emotional experience in pursuits of learning is a negative example of how collective accounts, themselves a kind of coalitional, situated knowledge, are always at work in our teaching spaces. We must be mindful of their lived presence and effects if we hope to change them—why I take the time here to explicitly recognize their deleterious effects.

I was reminded of the distance between our practice and our theory in a recent conversation with a colleague whom I believe is a very motivated and engaging teacher. As we shared tales of memorable classroom experiences, nostalgic at the end of yet another semester, my colleague noted that a student had recently cried in her presence. When I asked her how she responded, she looked genuinely confused and claimed that she "ignored it and did nothing" as if that were the only appropriate response available. Others on the periphery of our conversation nodded in a kind of compassionate agreement with her. This colleague seemed shocked to hear me tell stories of teaching encounters that validated and perhaps even encouraged student emotion, sharing moments when I hugged a student in distress and when I invited another student on the verge of tears over his lackluster performance on an essay and extenuating personal circumstances (his parents were divorcing) to my office to talk through his feelings and frustrations.

My colleague's surprise is understandable when placed against the larger backdrop of my department. Regularly included on the litany of instructors' complaints is students' insistence on bringing up their feelings in class. I hear often an echo of "I don't care what my students' feel; I just want them to think." When I hear this frustrated response, I must admit that I hear teachers' emotion, unacknowledged, short-circuiting valuable moments of potential learning so that rather than feeling empathy for the teacher, I tend to feel sympathy for students. It has always been curious to me how this complaint hides the ways students *are* articulating analytical thinking—using the language they have at hand, which often includes emotive discourse—but aren't being heard. Teachers' tend not to listen because of their own indoctrination in and gatekeeping of dominant pedagogies reliant on emotion's absent-presence, to borrow Worsham's language. Worsham argues that the absent-presence of feeling is perpetuated because we are taught a limited means of emotional expression and identification. Such silencing of emotion, guaranteed by our limited vocabulary, is a primary form of "pedagogic violence" meant to uphold the partriarchal status quo (Worsham, 2001, p. 240). Evoking the writing body, feelings become a "phantom limb" we must learn to suffer in silence (Worsham, 2001, pp. 247-251). The violence of a sundered limb highlights how we are unable to "adequately apprehend, name, and interpret [our] affective lives" and thus are left to view emotion as a private, dangerous and mysterious threat to public reason (Worsham, 2001, p. 240). The invited and critical expression of emotions is, then, an inherently a feminist endeavor and is fruitful ground for contemplative writing pedagogies.

But like the phantom limb that contradicts its non-presence when it tingles with pain, emotional expressions often do occur in our classrooms and offices, even if they are uninvited. I've heard colleagues label these moments as "outbursts," criticized on the grounds that they are only too telling of students' limited analytical powers, which makes students overly reliant on emotional cliché and performance. This pat response is best unpacked through Dawn Skorczewski's analysis of student writing, which investigates why students' beginning written discourse is often a hybrid blend of cliché and critical analysis. Cliché doesn't mean our students aren't thinking, Skorczewski claims as she examines student writing, only that they are using the ordinary language available to them to express those thoughts. Important to my analysis here, Skorczewski's notes that the clichés students use are often emotionally-loaded. Skorczewski's advice regarding teachers' reactions to student cliché might, in turn, be helpful to consider when approaching emotional discourse in our writing classes. Skorczewski's reminds us that "critical thought [may be] a kind of safe house for [teachers] in the same way that cliché can be for our students" (2000, p. 234). In other words, we judge our students' conceptions and expressions of their inner selves based on the ways we have ourselves been taught to mistrust personal and emotional language in favor of the discursive certainty of the poststructuralist self. As we acknowledge students' "lack of familiarity with how emotions work, we need to recall ways in which faculty embody or fail to embody critical emotional literacy as they situate themselves within the disciplinary culture of their fields" (Winans, 2012, p. 154). It would therefore be a greater critical (and feminist) gesture for us to revise our pedagogical rules and view awareness of our emotional positioning as a teachable skill in the writing classroom than for us to simply dismiss feeling altogether or write it off as clichéd and meaningless. Simply recognizing the flippant manner with which we approach student emotion is a step in the right direction: "the teacher who acknowledges the beliefs she brings to the conversation is equipped to listen to her students more carefully than the teacher who holds her beliefs so closely that she can no longer see them as beliefs" (Skorczewski, 2000, p. 236).

Here, following Skorczewski's gesture of rhetorical listening, I am interested in what changes when we begin to apply mindfulness to student emotion, viewing it not only as a readily-accessible discourse, as a feature of ordinary language, but also as a legitimate, embodied and critical engagement in the learning process—as a staple of the embodied imagination. In the next interchapter, I explore how contemplative pedagogy provides us a means of engaging student emotion and validating it as a generator of writing and meaning. When we begin to legitimate emotion, it seems to me that we open up our discussions of critical thinking to include feeling and thereby start to carve out new means of emotional expression, pulling it back into the ordinary language of classroom talk. Mindful discussion of emotion is necessary for us to create an environment where metacognition is a necessary and teachable feature of the writing process, as monitoring and controlling one's thoughts requires both motivation and continued effort, both of which are affective in nature. As Fleckenstein notes, we must talk to our students about how "much of writing consists of explosive moments of conflict … balanced—if we are lucky—by mystifying moments of flow" (1997, p. 28). In addition, we might also talk about the joy and pleasure of writing with our students. In the next section, I suggest that the concepts of "situated feeling" within contemplative writing pedagogy can help us perform this important work of recognizing the rhetorical and material effects of feeling.

SOLVING THE "PROBLEM" OF EMOTION THROUGH SITUATED FEELING

In Chapter Two, I treated situated knowing and feeling separately in order to develop a theory of situated knowledge for the feminist contemplative writing classroom; however, this separation is more reflective of the linear nature of a book than it is an indication of their status as separate faculties around which we can draw definitive lines. Contemplative approaches, in seeing education and learning as embodied, recognize that "full comprehension that arises as the fruit of contemplative pedagogy is not a remote, abstract, intellectual knowledge, but a form of beholding (theoria) that is fully embodied, which means that it entails aesthetic and moral dimensions as well as cognitive ones" (Zajonc, 2010, p. 91). To privilege the materiality of emotion as that which charges our flesh with agency, I move to define feeling in terms similar to those I used to define knowing in the last chapter. The overlap is unavoidable when we understand feeling and knowing as companion composers[20] of situated knowledge. If our knowledge is shaped just as much by our embodied feeling as our thinking, we must pay attention to both as creative forces in our writing. Building on Chapter Two's discussion of situated knowledge as that which gets made on the page and in the classroom in contemplative writing pedagogy, I am interested in seeing emotions as "situated feelings," marked by their corporeality as well as their social positioning, which creates and reflects the web of material situatedness from which we write. Parsing the definition of situated knowledge in light of this chapter's focus on emotion entails seeing situated knowledge as comprised of the two inexorably tied processes of situated thinking and situated feeling. An embrace of the material via this feminist contemplative epistemology brings the fleshy person back into view and testifies to her role in the construction of what is thought *and* felt. Situated feeling provides a theoretical model with which to counter the negative treatment of emotion in our lore-driven practices, as demonstrated in the last section, and a means of increasing our limited vocabulary of emotion in composition studies.

To review, Haraway defines situated knowledge as a feminist epistemology based on "particular and specific embodiment"[21] (1991c, p. 190) so that the body as an epistemic origin is seen to produce "partial, locatable, critical knowledge sustaining the possibility of webs of connection" in meaning making (1991c. p. 191). It is worth repeating the differences between understanding knowing and feeling through the lens of feminist situated knowledge as I do here instead of claiming a mainstream, postmodern situatedness, as has become routine among compositionists. As we've moved toward postmodern definitions of situatedness as the contingency surrounding all meaning, based on our placement in discursive systems that structure what and how we know, our pedagogies have typically closed out matter. Keeping a tension between mainstream constructivism and pedagogical alternatives, expressivists like Elbow and Lad Tobin have championed personal knowledge as a product of the individual in the world, but they tend to see this individual in terms of his/her psyche, too easily disconnecting the mind from the body.

Haraway's version of feminist situated knowledge deserves our attention for the ways it strikes a balance between pedagogies that rely too heavily on the exclusion of the "personal" for the social or vice versa, moving beyond inattention to the body. Situatedness from a Haraway-ian lens mediates: both the social construction of knowledge as well as the embodiment of our meaning making is taken into account. We aren't searching for the truth of the psyche or of the text but instead for responsible local knowledge that doesn't remove the knower from the known or cancel out the possibility of meaning outside the text. Attention to situatedness is meant to underscore just how central our embodied experience is; how knowledge, like the body, is always locatable and always partial. Indeed, situated knowledge rests on the subject's fleshiness, on her inherent embodiment as part of the organic world. Embodiment in this formulation takes on the meaning of "dynamically embedded" not "statically bound." Haraway defines situated knowledges as "marked knowledges" (1991c, p. 111) meaning that they are projects of knowing from the "somewhere" of the embodied subject as opposed to the "nowhere" of traditional empiricism or the "everywhere" of postmodernism (1991c, pp. 188-191). Alternately, Haraway advocates a strong embodiment in which the body is not just a window for knowing the world but is the map that structures our mapping of the world. We might even say that embodiment is knowing in this contemplative paradigm.

Embodiment is also feeling. The web-making process of situated knowing is one of "passionate construction" according to Haraway and "resonance, not … dichotomy" (1991c, pp. 194-195). As a critical and reflexive practice, situated knowledge thereby enacts what has been conventionally referred to as connected knowing in feminist literature. Sociologist Belenky defines connected knowing as "involv[ing] feeling, because it is rooted in relationship … [but also] involv[ing] thought" (Belenky, et al. 1973, p. 121). Because it invites feeling and sees emotion as critical and necessary to meaning, connected knowing advocates the epistemological stance of the "passionate knower" (1991c, p. 141). The passionate knower is a version of the embodied imaginer, or one engaged in situated knowing and feeling; one who is critical *and* emotional at the same time, recognizing that it is impossible to rise above the material self.

In exercising both mindfulness of her means of creating knowledge and the ways that knowledge ties her to others, the writer who takes on the role of embodied imaginer navigates a problem-solving context in which current emotional states, levels of motivation and perceptions of control are constantly being assessed through the introspective and reflective application of metacognition. The most recent educational research recognizes that affect and metacognition are bound together in much the same ways I am arguing that body and mind and feeling and knowing are linked in the contemplative. Preceding evaluative judgments of learning and knowing, "metacognitive feelings inform the person about a feature of cognitive processing, but they do it in an experiential way, that is, in the form of a feeling, such as feeling of knowing, feeling of confidence" (Efklides, 2006, p. 5). Writers who reflect on their learning between drafts of the same paper, for instance, do not do so in a cool and calculated way. They may ask themselves questions like, "How well am I understanding my audience's needs?", only to find that they are producing more writer-based than reader-based prose. Whether or not this becomes a moment of frustration and defeat in which the writer gives up or one of hopeful challenge in which the writer faces the problem with motivation and confidence in her ability to work through the recognized issue is feeling-laden. As I explore in the next interchapter, oftentimes, a writer's ability to be aware of her body's reaction to such a reflective process is key to her consciously processing the impact of her feelings on her writing process and using those feelings toward positive change and outcomes. As I will show there, if she can use her breath to work through the tensions of problem-solving, she may perceive her control of the situation to be greater than if she is unaware of this embodied tension.

Here, I'd like to focus on how the embodied imaginer, who understands meaning-making through the lens of situated knowledge, is summarily engaged in a process of situated thinking *and* feeling. In this contemplative process, it is understood that:

- Feeling is seen as an agentive force of the body, not simply a rhetorical construct and therefore not entirely reducible to language even if it is reciprocally shaped by it.
- The body is the origin of both feeling as well as thinking. Both processes must be interwoven to create responsible, local knowledge.
- Our understanding of feeling is primarily experiential but our common embodiment, which can be seen as a promising and productive "limitation," produces certain schemas of emotion that are shared so that we can connect to others. Thus, it makes sense to talk about the interaction of bodies and cultures wherein both shape each other.
- Situated feeling establishes a "webbed" orientation that allows for the creation of connected knowledge, which rejects traditional modes of detachment and seeks to relate the material and discursive at the level of meaning and enact it at the level of our bodies.
- As such, situated feeling prompts one to understand one's limits and one's partial perspective, encouraging a recognition of embodied difference and the need to build coalitions among others differentially positioned.

As these five central premises of situated feeling show, definitions of situated knowledge from the last chapter are not balanced unless they account for the enmeshment of feeling and thinking. Situated knowledges are, in part, marked by feeling since they both place us in a material body and spatialize us in the world. Situated feeling highlights the ways materiality and discursivity are yoked in circles of meaning, making it impossible and particularly senseless to separate them. We are left, then, with a view of emotion as equally embedded in the organic body as in culture, or as situated in both material and semiotic worlds. Viewing emotion through situated feeling necessitates that we give up the closure of defining it as entirely linguistic or natural. It similarly hampers any attempts to define emotion, feeling, or affect separately, encouraging my interchangeable use of these terms.

I choose "situated feeling" instead of alternatives like Laura Micciche's more performative "rhetorics of emotion" (2007) because the latter too often establishes the body as a discursive marker, denying its agentive materiality. Despite a weaker focus on the body than I am calling for, Micciche has done much recent work in composition studies to make emotions visible and intelligible, and her book *Doing Emotion: Rhetoric, Writing, Teaching* makes as an exciting counterstatement to a mainstream alignment of emotion with persuasive, pathetic appeals in line with classical rhetoric's valuative positioning of *pathos* beneath *logos* and *ethos*—despite its seeming equal weight among the rhetorical appeals. Aligning emotion with a social sense of "doing" leads Micciche to differentiate "emoting," which she defines as the individual expression of feeling, from "rhetorics of emotion," or "emotion as a performative that produces effects. To speak of emotion as performative is to foreground the idea that emotions are enacted and embodied in the social world … [and that] we *do* emotions—they don't simply happen to us" (2007, pp. 1-2). It is with the latter, the doing of emotion, that Micciche is concerned.

Micciche's work raises fruitful questions about how contemplative writing pedagogies might take up the meaning-making potential of situated feeling. While not aligning her work with embodiment as directly as I am, Micciche acknowledges the connection between research on emotion and the body, citing neurobiological evidence that we come to know our emotions by the ways in which we embody and experience them (2007, p. 19). Research on both bodies and feelings therefore often share similar exigencies. Consequently, what binds Micciche's and my undertaking of emotion is the need to address emotion's fullness, seeing it not simply as a way to move an audience (a persuasive aim) but also as a dynamic motor of meaning (a generative process). When viewed as a situated act, emotion's meaning and value for writing need not be understood in a strictly personal sense, and it can therefore be understood as teachable and necessary for critical narratives and metacognitive insight.

Micciche is as resistant to understanding emotion simply as a quality of the private mind as I am, since it is this kind of "commonsense" view that has led to emotion's devaluation. For this author, our understanding of emoting as an ineffable, private expression of feeling has blinded us to the relational conception of emotion as circulation. It is the concept of emotion as private that propels the lore evident in the personal example I used to frame this chapter and leads Bartholomae to argue that expressivism, the pedagogy historically most aligned with the validation of feeling in writing, promotes sentimental realism by encouraging writers to see their compositions as "true stor[ies] of what [they] think, feel, know and see" (1990, p. 69).[22] Whether or not the body is our focus, we must begin to see feeling as both social and personal if we wish to reanimate our studies of it and hope for its inclusion in our pedagogies.

Micciche understands emotions as "emerging relationally, in encounters between people, so that emotion takes form between bodies rather than residing in them" (2007, p. 13). A relational, constitutive understanding of emotion underscores it as a rhetorical "technology for doing" (2007, p. 14) as opposed to a private reaction or a persuasive tool for consumption and not production.

Micciche uses the view of emotion as circulation, "emotion takes form between bodies rather than residing in them" (2007, p. 13) to avoid the privatization of emotion that constructivists target. Resisting the view of emotions as tools used to manipulate reason, Micciche instead forwards a notion of emotions as constructive *acts* of meaning by drawing from Sarah Amhed's work on emotions in politics.

To understand what sets Micciche's approach apart from the classical canon of work on emotion, the distinction to press is the way emotions are here seen as always present, acting as constructors of meaning by binding individuals together in economies of value. Emotions, as such, are not simply passive tools of provocation. We cannot choose to "add in" emotions since they are always already present making meaning and shaping values, bodies and beliefs—whether or not we attend to these dynamics. For her, what we have failed to see is how the *performance* of emotion is what connects individuals in social groups, making feelings powerful measures of group realities. Micciche calls the effects of emotion's relational circulation "stickiness" after Ahmed. Stickiness accounts for the ways signs are positioned as objects of feeling so that they accumulate specific, affective values which attach to them through narratives and discursive structures like metaphor (2007, p. 27). The term takes on a webbing conception connecting the individual who feels to a larger network of material subjects and objects by the web-spinning of language as it works like a spider.

I have no desire to argue against the social construction of emotion or to conceive of emotion as ineffable, since I am working within a model of situatedness myself, but Micciche's primary focus on the social body over the individual body marks the point at which our approaches diverge as she goes to rhetorics of emotion and I to situated feeling. In making the claim of sticky relationality within rhetorics of emotion, Micciche strives to underscore the ways in which we perform feelings based on certain cultural scripts or feeling rules and casts her lot with the group over the individual per se. For her, the performance of emotion as socially saturated is where the hope for transformation lies. This is plainly evident in Micciche's instructive example of how emotions bind together individuals into a social body when she turns to the ways composition's identity metaphors attach particular emotional valences to the field.

In particular, Micciche explores the negative emotions of subjection, what Wendy Brown calls a "wound culture," as that which binds together the theory, the practice and the teachers within composition (2007, p. 28). Micciche's point is that composition's emotioned response, which is a central feature of its rhetoric of subjection, reproduces its marginalization in a cycle that might be understood as a self-fulfilling prophecy. To break this destructive cycle, Micciche claims we need a new emotional identity for our field and offers the process model of "performative composition" which derives from Butler's notion of gender as a repeated performance of "stylized acts" which solidify into an identity that seems natural (2007, p. 44).

Micciche's stake in the performance of emotion takes its cue from Butler's definition of gender. For Butler, gender is "*a corporeal style*, an 'act,' as it were, which is both intentional and performative, where '*performative*' suggests a dramatic and contingent construction of meaning" (1999, p. 177). Gender is not "in" us but is rather an externalized effect: "There is no gender identity behind the expressions of gender; that identity is performatively constituted by the very "expressions" that are said to be its results" (1999, p. 33). If, like our gender identity, composition's identity as wounded only *appears* innate, but is rather naturalized through certain performances, there is room to remake the field and thereby invite new performances and positive understandings of its emotional culture. Through our emotions, compositionists have the power to adhere to the affective status quo or to take action and reenergize our emotional metaphors, thereby changing the social dynamics of the field. The bulk of Micciche's book consequently focuses on composition's current emotional culture and the ways in which it can be re-envisioned, offering much constructive criticism along the way.

However, as I explored in Chapter One, when Butler extends her performance theory to sex, the body becomes a sign emptied of its materiality.[23] To testify to the social construction of sex, Butler encourages us to see matter as "*a process of materialization that stabilizes over time to produce the effect of boundary, fixity and surface*" (1993, p. 26). The body therefore becomes more a sign or "effect" than a real physical presence. While I share Micciche's desire to move from a cognitive model of emotion as interiority, I believe shifting to exteriority disallows the body's hold on emotion and thus devalues situated feeling as I have defined it. Within feminism, I go to Haraway precisely because she refuses to etherealize the body. Even if we read Micciche generously so that the body does not entirely disappear, it does seem to acquire the status of yet another "object of feeling" that *accumulates* sticky affect rather than *produces* it, so that the body is often better understood as a stage for the performance than an agent of it.

So while I find useful her conceptualization of emotion as sticky circulation, the trouble spot for me in Micciche's definition of emotion is the binary established by her placement of "rather:" again, "emotion takes form between bodies *rather* than residing in them" (2007, p. 13, emphasis added). This binary is reflected in her desire to divorce emoting from rhetorics of emotion, a division I find unnecessary since there is no analytic of emotion, no performance of feeling, without individual bodies emoting; the personal body's expression and shaping of feeling must occur within rhetorics of emotion or we would have nothing to analyze since our linguistic and conceptual schemas of emotion most certainly rest on our physical experiences of them. Situated feeling, as I have conceived of it with Haraway's help, provides an alternative that generates a fuller analytic of feeling, which sees emotion as residing in bodies as well as moving between and among them. In sum, it recaptures the presence of the contemplative writing body, the writing yogi, a term I fully explain in Chapter One.

Placing emotion only between bodies may work to uncover a construction of affective meaning in social groups like the discipline of composition studies, but it seems less helpful in developing a praxis of contemplative writing wherein the individual expression of situated writing bodies is equally as important to the making and exploration of meaning through composing as it is to understanding collective, affective economies in the classroom. Micciche's focus on the top-down circulation of emotion may avoid the essentialist charge, but it also seems to place more emphasis on discursive, rhetorical movement than sticky bodies as agents of rhetoric themselves. For instance, the emphasis on social bodies overagainst individual bodies, which rhetorizes rather than actualizes flesh, is supported by Micciche's proposed classroom activities such as when students are asked to read and record a section of a teacher-chosen text where emotioned language seems present. Students then record and perform this section for classmates, opening class dialogue on the movement of emotion, thereby unearthing the stickiness of emotion as it pulses through texts and between the bodies of writers, readers and audiences at large (Micciche, 2007, p. 58).[24]

What this activity teaches students about the construction of identity in the production of emotion is certainly valuable, but the student's own writing body, her feeling center, seems lost here for the performance of the author's. Rather than using only the projected personae of authors, in contemplative pedagogy, students would be just as likely to read their own written texts. Such reading could lead to productive discussions about how emotion is flexibly situated depending on the reading and the reception of a text. This practice could show how our reading is also contingent on the emotion that "stuck" to the original composition by the way of style, tone, language and even the embodied memory of the writing to which the author is privy; it might also reveal an unexpected disruption, creating emotional dissonance for the author of the text which may or may not be felt by other readers. Another option might be for us to engage students in an embodied and experiential analysis of their emotions as they relate to their understanding of how their writing selves are created. Amy

Winans describes a potential activity in her article advocating contemplative pedagogies within literature classes that engage students in an examination of difference and a questioning of privilege. Indeed, she argues that we must attend to emotional literacy if we ask students to confront difference in our courses. Winans sees contemplative practice as a means of engaging students in analytical and experiential engagements with their emotions toward the end of developing critical emotional awareness (2012, p. 152). Winans asks students to "spend ten minutes outside of class standing in a public place doing nothing—without pretending to be doing something (waiting, checking a phone, people watching, looking for something" and to write a paper about that experience (2012, p. 160). This contemplative activity is meant to promote students' analysis of silence and any emotions of discomfort caused by engaging directly in experience without distraction. Winans concludes that such contemplative practice both allows students to feel the way their identity shifts in their interactions (or lack thereof) with others and also how their bodies are implicated in emotional responses. With this recognition comes the responsibility to analyze emotions that result from habitual thinking and the responsibility to recognize how our emotional states can impact the ways we can make and interpret meaning from experience (Winans, 2012, p. 161). Contemplative exercises like these can show students that there is movement and stickiness in situated feeling but that there are also times of dynamic rest in positioned bodies; that feeling isn't just *in* language, it is also *in* bodies.

To argue for both is in line with contemplative embodiment. Contemplative philosophy and feminist theory together provide us a theory of situated knowledge in which the body is not just a stage on which cultural scripts like gender are played but is more like a sage actor who improvises as much as she follows a script, changing the play as it unfolds. By adding situated feeling to this theory, we can see that we simply could not conceive of emotions if we did not first perceive them as residing inside us and as essential to the ways in which our fleshy bodies navigate the world. Our experiences of embodiment include both interiority and exteriority, reminding us that feelings can be viewed as part of the body's extralingustic agency without negating the role our culture has to play in our shaping. Recognizing the body's role encourages us to learn to develop an awareness that speaks *with* the body and not always *for* it.

BRINGING THEORY TO PRACTICE: SITUATED FEELING THROUGH EMOTIONAL FLEXIBILITY

Western conceptions of the body have tended toward devaluation and dismissal of our flesh. However, Eastern practices are able to sustain the development of such somatic awareness where our own cultural practices may fall short. Yoga, like composition, is at its heart, a praxis or an applied philosophy. Because it is a practice of doing, one that enforces process and practice just as writing does, yoga harmonizes well with the tenor of writing rhetorics. What may matter most to contemplative writing pedagogies is that yoga also takes the body as an epistemic origin so that embodiment becomes the means of knowing, feeling and making sense of the world and not just a physical enactment of social forces. Locating ourselves in our bodies, or developing a corporeal orientation that can translate to our writing, is a skill useful on the mat and in the classroom. A corporeal orientation insists on viewing knowledge as situated and therefore suggests that just as we are positioned by our material situatedness, the places and spaces our bodies occupy, we are positioned also by our feelings, which can be seen as negotiations between the agency of our bodies and the social circulation of affect in society. Yoga recognizes not only the theory but also the practice of situated knowing and feeling.

As I explored in my first and second interchapters, the practice of yoga can provide compositionists new theoretical lenses and practical methods to teach students how to create an embodied writing process. My central premise there was that yoga can show students on both a metaphorical level as well as an embodied, pragmatic one that our materiality helps shape the meaning we make in our writing. It follows that body awareness is a skill that can lead to more successful and generative writing sessions as well as a deeper understanding of the meaning-making process. And while I could potentially follow any contemplative practice to develop my argument, I concentrate on Iyengar yoga, a branch of Hatha, because of my experience with it and because of its core value of adaptability based on student needs and abilities.

I've argued that feminist contemplative writing pedagogies engage in a feminist epistemology of situated thinking and feeling. These pedagogies are consequently invested in getting students to practice connected knowing, a mode of knowing that is personal even when the object of knowing is not (Belenky, et al., 1973, p. 21). In contrast to separate knowers who experience the self as autonomous, connected knowers experience the self as always in a webbed relation to the material world and to others. Yoga theory and practice ultimately follows a similar connective impulse: it seeks balance and integration; it recognizes difference but does not see it as divisive. When placed within embodied writing pedagogy, the knowing facilitated by yoga can be seen to result in the formation of connected, situated knowledge that sees diversity as a generative force balanced by a commonality of flesh. Our bodies literally and conceptually provide the structure for the awareness, respect and mediation of difference.

Part of this awareness entails being receptive to our and others' situated feelings, which is a skill teachable in the writing classroom and necessary for students' lives outside of it. Far from promoting solipsism, attending to situated feeling attunes us to others and to the outside world of matter as it underscores the physicality of our knowing processes and the idea that understanding is itself material, not simply cerebral, in nature. Rooted in our bodies, we are also connected to other forms of matter. Calling to mind many of yoga's themes of interconnectedness, philosopher Richard Shusterman argues that we feel our bodies in relation to other bodies of matter:

> One cannot really feel oneself somatically without also feeling something of the external world. If I lie down, close my eyes, and carefully try to feel just my body in itself, I will also feel the way it makes contact with the floor and sense the space between my limbs. (2008, p. 70)

Of course, the practice of *asana* asks us to make sense of these feelings, both sensational and emotional, in order to better understand ourselves and the world in which we live. In my yoga class, these feelings also help build a sense of community that links together individual bodies as we move and breathe in harmony, often unconsciously synchronizing our actions and drawing a sense of strength and solidarity from each other even as we move through *asanas* on our own mats. Linda Adler-Kassner sees the potential of yoga to teach writers and program administrators the importance of communing with others in her 2008 book, *The Activist WPA*. Using her experience as a yoga student, Adler-Kassner argues that yoga teaches that "[o]ur breath is our own, yes. But when we hear the breath of others and develop our practice in concert with others, that practice changes in ways we don't always anticipate" (Adler-Kassner, 2008, p. vii). Together, these ideas testify that a turn to the self does not close out others, but can indeed make us more aware of our relatedness to the larger world of matter.

My experiences as a yogi suggest how I might bring such a focus on situated feeling into my writing classrooms. Using yoga as a creative guide, I'd like to suggest a pragmatic approach to attend to situated feelings within contemplative writing pedagogy, one that provides a positive hermeneutic and gives viability to their instructional inclusion. I argue that we should strive to teach our students emotional flexibility, or to be yogis of their emotions, in order to engage them in producing the thinking and feeling processes that will lead to situated knowledge. Doing so affords students the agency to negotiate their embodied realities in relation to the reflective discourse on experience we encourage them to develop as part of the process of critical analysis. It stands opposed to asking them to somehow transcend these realities for the sake of a disembodied textual-social analysis or simple appropriation of a new discourse community. Emotional flexibility is part of a feminist process of critical engagement and inquiry that does not cancel out feeling and focuses on a holistic notion of "critical being" rather than simply critical thinking. In working through a new notion of emotion through flexibility, I am hoping to address the problem Worsham articulates in Going Postal, that we will continue to struggle with emotion's inclusion in our pedagogies until we refuse to allow it to remain "beyond our semantic availability" (2001, p. 240). A contemplative means of talking about emotion may just give us the impetus to work through its effects in our classrooms and a language to share with our students. If situated feeling can help guide our theories, emotional flexibility can gives us a means of talking about emotion in the classroom.

Developing Flexibility on the Mat

In his definitive book on yoga, *Light on Life*, Iyengar targets two complementary skills necessary for the development of flexibility through the practice of *asanas* or poses: "extension," attending to our inner space, and "expansion," reaching out toward others and the unknown beyond us. Both acts are situated within a personal body but teach this body simultaneously to be inner-directed and outer-directed. Extension and expansion are interrelated actions because to reach out and create new space, you must first understand your own locatedness, or be aware of your center—what we might otherwise call our situatedness in a particular body in the world. Extension is attention to our immediate space, focusing on being *in* the personal body. Actions of extension include centering oneself through reflection and developing awareness of one's thoughts and feelings. In other words, this skill includes reflection on the processes of situated knowing and engaging in situated feeling, actions which insist on a personal attentiveness that joins the "sensitive awareness of the body and the intelligence of the brain and heart ... [together] in harmony" (Iyengar, 2005, p. 29). Extension asks us to marry the thinking and feeling postures that permeate the doing of a pose and is practiced attentively when both means of expression are balanced. Feeling in this equation may be understood as, in part, sensational, a slowing heartbeat and steady hands, as well as emotive and conceptual, such as feelings of peacefulness and receptivity.

While vision isn't unimportant here, it does get dethroned from its typical position of authority since yoga recognizes the limitations of sight. Increasing flexibility through awareness "is different from seeing with your normal two eyes. Instead you are feeling; you are sensing the position of your body" (Iyengar, 2005, p. 29). Feeling can indeed be more powerful than sight because it exchanges the receptivity of two outward-looking eyes for the awareness of the entire sensitive body which folds in on itself (through extension) as well as out toward the world (through expansion).[25] When practicing warrior III, for instance, I cannot see the leg I lift behind me as my body leans forward and I balance on the other leg; nor can I always see if my outstretched arms are parallel to the floor—if I try to look behind me, I lose my balance. Instead, I must learn through practice to feel the positioning of my leg behind me and to use my feelings as a guide to how to maneuver my body in space. To find balance, I need to be aware of the sensations of the pose, the emotions the pose calls up and the ways my intellect processes this bodily input and language captures and shapes it. It's a bridging of body, brain and heart so that I experience myself as dynamically rooted, since the means of this bridging changes moment-by-moment as I take in the outside world with my in-breath and release with my out-breath. The acts of extension root us in the personal body, helping us understand our immediate material-semiotic placement and provide a path toward self-determination, but they are not to be completed alone.

Expansion complements extension because it reaches beyond the self's perceived center. The body unfolds and energy flows outward. Actions of expansion include the experience of creating spaces in new directions; an opening of the inner body and expanding to the experience of the external. Using a concrete example of expansion to show how it works together with extension to promote awareness and increase flexibility, Iyengar states, "When most people stretch, they simply stretch *to* the point they are trying to reach, but they forget to extend and expand from where they are. When you expand and extend, you are not only stretching *to*, you are also stretching *from*. Try holding out your arm at your side and stretch it. Did your whole chest move with it? Now try to stay centered and extend out your arm to your fingertips .... Did you notice the space you created and the way in which you stretched from your core?" (Iyengar, 2005, pp. *Light* 33-34). I invite my reader to try this exercise. The space created through this stretching is the space for new ideas and transgressed boundaries. We experience our limits differently when we expand; for when we only extend, we may feel limited by the length of our grasp. But, when we also expand, we recognize that we can stretch out much further than we first thought; we create new openness. As this simple exercise shows, we actually create more space by being aware of our bodies and centered in them as opposed to simply reaching out with no thought as to the embodied origin of that movement.

In warrior III, expansion encourages me to reach my leg out from the center of my body, but extension reminds me to ground the stretch in the resistance I create by pressing my tailbone into my pelvis instead of reaching my arms out as far forward as possible. A lesson I relearn each time I practice is that mindlessly reaching out without conscious extension will push too much weight on the ball of my standing foot and not enough on my heel, making me tip forward. Without a balanced sense of self, I cannot reach toward the unknown. Instead, I must feel my arms create space against the resisting pull of my leg in the opposite direction as if I were pinching a rubber band with two fingers and attending to those fingers as much as the feeling of pulling the rubber band in the opposite direction. This pose makes me understand the importance of feeling centered in my hips and middle body so that I can reach beyond the center without losing myself for the sake of the movement itself; it's a conscious action. Attentive form makes this pose a freeing experience at the same time as a rooted one, dependent quite literally on the stability of my standing leg as if it were a tree trunk sinking roots into the earth—an imaginative visualization I often use. Literally and metaphorically, this kind of movement increases flexibility at the same time that it demands we remain accountable to the limits of our flesh.

Emotional Flexibility in the Classroom

Extension and expansion are useful terms to use when working through the kind of emotional flexibility we might guide our students to develop as part of the embodied rhetorical process of contemplative knowing. Teaching emotional extension would entail helping students extend awareness to their emotional states as they write and the ways in which their bodies speak through their feelings. Students can be guided to articulate their situated feelings and the personal knowledge that has been shaped by and helped to shape those feelings in turn. In my classes, I've used reflective blogs as low-stakes journaling spaces wherein students can express their feelings and explore them in relation to what we are learning in class as well as the meaning they create through their writing. I also ask them to reflect on the emotional endeavor of the writing process itself, encouraging them to metacognitive insight. As I detailed in an earlier chapter, completing a regular *asana* practice as part of the composing process itself helps students tune into their feelings, sensational and emotional, in order to garner a better sense of what they take into their writing and how certain topics may incite feeling responses that they pass on to the page. These actions of turning in do not encourage self-centeredness. Reflection on personal emotional states develops flexibility and not simple solipsism because students can learn to move beyond crippling self-consciousness and concentrate on exploring how they feel and not what others might be thinking or how they believe they should feel. This validates students, giving them agency to make sense of their experiences in light of others' and guarantees a rhetorical process invested in the creation of new knowledge and not an exploration of already-formed ideas by published authors, experts.

It is precisely this agentive impulse that generates Hindman's argument in Making Writing Matter wherein she argues against the theoretical status quo that insists our rhetorical realties are more important or genuine than our embodied realities. In this article, Hindman uses her own lived experience as an alcoholic to argue against such already-formed "expert" ideas that our identities are ideological constructions that interpolate us into certain master narratives. Instead, she insists she is unwilling to transcend the body she knows has a reality outside of discourse; that the rhetoric of alcoholism helped to define an embodied reality she was living long before she ever stepped foot into an AA meeting and began to accept their language of recovery. Hindman concedes that when she constructs herself as an alcoholic, she is submitting herself to a discourse, but she argues that this is an empowering choice, or a "way I could hope to escape the deterministic and bleak physical aspects" of being an alcoholic (2001, p. 99). In other words, in choosing to control what it means to be an alcoholic and taking the language that labels to make it enable, Hindman creates a kind of embodied agency within language. Her body is a source of agency and power, allowing her to escape the dominant yet negative understanding of alcoholism and to recognize the role of her flesh in making meaning and, especially in this case, in the process of revision (ie., her revision of the alcoholic's identity narrative). To the extent that we see our own students as "recovering alcoholics" who abuse the comforts of the status quo by ignoring the ways in which they might be interpolated by their cultures and societies and relying too heavily on emotional discourse as opposed to alcohol, we may treat them as Hindman fears: as pawns of ideology who need to be taught to appropriate the theories of experts in order to complete smart social analysis. Incorporating attention to extension may encourage students' development of an emotional flexibility that validates their embodied feelings. In turn, they can enter into discourse communities as bodies with resistances, the first of which is feeling itself.

Even so, to balance this act of understanding feeling as residing in us, as a part of our corporeal fabric as embodied beings, we also need to teach students to see emotion as that which connects them to social structures, or how affect works *in between* cultures and individuals in addition to *within* individuals. That is, how feeling spatializes our body in relation to other bodies in the world by web-making through connections. As a result, feeling is a tangible way to localize our knowledge-making practices. When we see feeling as an enabling marker of local knowledge, we attend to how our affective relations to the world are mapping practices that materialize in the social interactions of bodies, which disturbs easy categories of private and public and inner and outer. In turn, we begin to respect the ways we should accept the openness of their definitions, refusing hard and fast delineations between the two. Finding comfort in closure is an act of unbendingness or inflexibility.

Emotional expansion is useful here because it pushes us out in new, sometimes uncomfortable ways and gives us means to see how the social circulation of emotion between bodies works. We must give up control, to prompt a flexibility of thinking and feeling with others and beyond the insular self. Vulnerability becomes strength for those who reach out and increased self-awareness is often an unexpected outcome. Famous yoga instructor Rodney Lee states this eloquently saying, "I believe we're doing yoga so that we can be strong enough to be fragile …. I don't think yoga is to keep you from feeling fragile. I think it's to enable you to be consciously fragile but still feel like, 'I'm fine with this fragility'" (2002, p. 4). Teaching students to consider seriously their classmates' ideas helps to achieve this end. I've had students practice contemplative listening in written responses to peers who disagreed with their ideas, asking them to write back to their peer in ways that attempted to respect the dissension and work with it as opposed to simply negate it. Even more than such strategies alone, introducing the embodied imagination as a method for the process of inquiry in composition studies, one that takes its lineage from feminism and an Eastern tradition of yoga that challenges hierarchical dualities and seeks integration at its core, may show students how to stretch themselves without denying or hurting their embodied selves in the process. I enflesh the contemplative theory of situated feeling presented here in the next interchapter by exploring how it translates to the classroom and gives meaning to a practice of breath control, or *pranayama*, in the contemplative writing classroom.

INTERCHAPTER THREE:[26] THE WRITER'S BREATH

> Your practice is your laboratory.
> —BKS Iyengar, *Light on Life*

> Om, shanti, shanti, shanti. (Om, peace, peace, peace)
> —yoga mantra

> To grow as a writer is to grow as a person.
> —Student

"Alright, everyone knows what to do," I say. "Be sure to sit up straight in your chair and plant your feet firmly on the ground, letting that connection give you a sense of stability and rootedness, like how you feel in tree pose." Some students shift with these words, but many remain still, already practicing the attentiveness we've been cultivating over the past few weeks. They have learned that being relaxed and being attentive are not separate states but can be coupled for greater awareness, and they are using their bodies to achieve this harmony.

"Now, softly close your eyes," I tell them, noting with pleasure that a handful of students had closed their eyes well before my verbal prompt. "Bring the lids together, touching but not squeezing them, so you feel the horizon of your sealed eyelids.[27] With this action, let the pupils of your eyes begin to migrate slowly toward the back of your head. Feel the release that gives you in your forehead."[28] I look out and see my twenty writing students with their eyes closed, waiting patiently for my next verbal cue to continue our classroom practice of mindful breathing, also known as *pranayama* in the tradition of Iyengar yoga.

"Scan your body for tension and release it. Allow your shoulders to drop away from your neck and observe your tongue. If it is pressed up onto the roof of your mouth, relax it down onto the floor of your mouth. Let the inner walls of your throat soften and spread away from one another, so you feel the hallway of your throat becoming wider and wider. Tune your ears inward, and begin to listen to the sound of your own breath." For a few moments, I pause to relax and listen to my inhalations and exhalations, collecting my thoughts and readying myself for today's lesson and our imminent class discussion. With some effort, I let go of everything beyond the present moment of sitting in front of this class, my eyes closed, breathing with my students. As I hear our breaths mingle, I feel bonded to my students and peaceful, removed from the rush of morning meetings and lesson planning that began my day.

"Pay attention to your breath, the inhalations and the exhalations, without trying to change them," I say after a long pause without opening my eyes. "Now, based on how you are feeling today, choose which breath is right for you. If you are tired, work on our three-part inhalation, sharply inhaling to your lower, middle, then upper ribs. Pause after each inhale and once you reach the top ribs, release your breath in a steady exhale. If you are stressed and anxious, begin to deepen your exhalations, so they become longer than your inhalations. See your inhalations as "small" and your exhalations as "big." You can try inhaling for three slow counts and exhaling for five slow counts, if this helps. If you are feeling fairly balanced already, simply concentrate on smoothing out your inhalations and exhalations, making them soft and quiet."

"Allow your inhalations to give you energy and your exhalations to expel all the worries and stresses of your day. Find peace in your breath." I look for peace in my own breath as I give students a few moments to find a similar calm in themselves before guiding us back to regular breathing. "Let your breathing return to normal, but keep it smooth and calm. Keeping your eyes closed, pay attention to your feelings of peace, awareness and steadiness. Resolve to carry these into the rest of your day. The peace you feel now is yours to return to at any point; you just have to remember it and work toward it once again. Similarly, if you have found focus and awareness now, you can find them again within."

I end the breathing exercise by asking my students to invoke a goal they are ready to embody: "Now, take a minute to set an intention for yourself. Your intention could be grounded in the learning goals you have for our class or for all of your classes. It may even encompass your social and academic lives. What do you hope to accomplish today or this week as a writer and a learner?" I am silent as I set my own intention and let students set theirs.

"Now that you have set it, remember to revisit your intention later today and later this week. Use it as a guide for your behavior and a checkpoint for yourself. When you are ready, slowly open your eyes." I ask my students to freewrite for a few minutes as a way to continue our observation of quiet mindfulness and to begin directly applying it to our writing. In her freewrite, Megan questions the form of her developing essay on body image dilemmas for young, female athletes; she isn't happy with the argument she has produced. She writes of her intention to listen to her "gut" regarding what changes she needs to make to her essay's form instead of too easily allowing other readers to sway her choices, a problem she has documented before. Johnny sets an intention to find a central focus to his wandering thoughts, to put them "inside one of these focused breaths," and Adam promises himself the freedom to explore his ideas instead of just sticking with the first one he has. Adam notes that this is a social goal too since he tends to be stubborn in his writing as well as in his daily living. After a moment to find our voices, we begin the day's lesson with renewed energy and focus, plunging into our classroom work with mindfulness.

HARMONIZING BREATHING AND WRITING

I share a version of guided *pranayama*—the Sanskrit term for our meditative, focused breathing practice—I've used in my writing courses in order to provoke new ideas about how we might engage students' writing bodies in our classes and attend to the meaning potential of feeling. Western conceptions of the body have often devalued and dismissed our feeling flesh. Tompkins' early call in Me and My Shadow to embrace the personal and embodied dimensions of our writing and her entreaty for us to give up the pretense of the disembodied and impersonal voice in our writing and accept the real body, "the human frailty of the speaker … his emotions, his history" that supports the writing persona as well as the "moment of intercourse with the reader—acknowledgement of the other person's presence, feelings, needs" (1987, p. 175) have since led to treatises on embodied pedagogy, including Hindman's Making Writing Matter and, recently, Kazan's Dancing Bodies in the Classroom and Fleckenstein's *Embodied Literacies*. Recent attempts to consider the writer's materiality haven't always taken a global perspective, however, and have consequently remained silent on one of the most viable ways of attending to the somatics of learning and the physicality of writing: contemplative education. Drawing on an over 2,500 year-old history of Eastern contemplative traditions, contemplative education approaches the learner holistically, as a body-heart-mind, and utilizes contemplative practice to transform traditional curricula. As such, contemplative pedagogies offer writing studies concrete methods of engaging the body in education and a means of developing writers' mindful awareness of themselves and others as I assert in previous chapters. Because of their ability to help students become contextual thinker-actors and creative global citizens, contemplative approaches to learning are rapidly growing in higher education (see, for instance, Simmer-Brown & Grace, 2011).

In our own field, Moffett was an early adopter of contemplative education, before it was even labeled as such, when he argued that "[w]riting and meditating are naturally allied activities" (1982, p. 231). Despite growing academic interest in contemplative education, few within writing studies have followed Moffett's early inquiries, even as university culture becomes more and more permeated by contemplative practice and education, what Zajonc calls the "silent revolution" of higher education (2010, p. 91). This book has been organized around an effort to explore what kind of revolution contemplative education might bring to writing studies. As I have outlined it, this so-called revolution might be summed up by the term I coined in my introduction to explain the shift that occurs when we ask students to engage in contemplative pedagogies: the embodied imagination. I have highlighted the consequences of becoming embodied imaginers in my chapters as I explored how we might help students reclaim the meaning-making potential of their bodies in both Chapter and Interchapter One. In the second interchapter and chapter pair, I argued that seeing writing as an embodied process and approaching student writers as writing yogis means that we must approach the learning process differently too, and that conceptions of situated knowledge can help us to do so. Not only does situated knowledge shift our thinking from personal/social binaries to a more inclusive and connected picture of knowledge-making, it also helps us respect the qualities of transformative openness and metacognitive insight developed by contemplative learning and knowing. In this final interchapter, I will conclude my exploration of the embodied imagination as a product of contemplative pedagogy by continuing what I started in Chapter Three: looking at how the embodied heuristic of feeling can help students become more reflective and generative writers.

As I've noted earlier, while I could go to any contemplative tradition to transform my classes, I have chosen to use yoga to help teach my students rhetorical awareness and mindfulness of living and learning. It is a commonplace among contemplative educators that individual instructors must choose the practices that guide our pedagogies based on our own practices and interests. My opening points to the ways I intend to use this chapter to further explore an integrated yoga-writing pedagogy that teaches students to embody the writing process with the breath. I am drawn to yoga (which includes the exercises of postures, meditation, and focused, meditative breathing), because it is, like composition, a praxis or an applied philosophy. Because it is a practice of doing, much like writing, yoga harmonizes well with the tenor of writing rhetorics. From this convergence, I will argue that developing writers' "emotional flexibility" by teaching them to engage their feeling bodies through the practice of *pranayama*, or meditative, controlled breathing, can not only enrich their felt experience of the writing process and the physical ease and comfort with which they write but can also attune them to the materiality of knowledge making. Students who use *pranayama* as a regular composing ritual begin to appreciate the body as a site of learning and understand writing as a somatic experience that occurs with and through the flesh.

I will explore how students who self-consciously engage in these embodied writing practices develop, in turn, a greater metacognitive awareness of the writing process, reflected in their writings *about* writing. "Contemplative practices are metacognitive attention-training ... research on learning establishes that since meditation is metacognitive it supports ideal learning" (Repetti, 2010, p. 13). Since yoga promotes metacognition, it follows that dramatic gains can be seen in writing yogi's writing about writing, a space ripe for the display of their thinking and reflecting. In other words, as students breathe their way into writing, they place new value on observing the writing process as it unfolds, documenting and analyzing the felt experience of composing, which helps them become more generative and reflective writers. Particularly, students' increased mindfulness and flexibility results in developed focus and advanced coping mechanisms to deal with the negative emotions of the writing process. Because these emotions are most likely to shut down the writing process and encourage our students' procrastination, which can hinder the development of their thinking and their drafts, we have a responsibility to attend to student emotion in our classrooms, as I argued in Chapter Three.

To give sufficient space to students' vocalizations of their feeling bodies, as represented in the reflective, metacognitive writings they produced during our class, like my other two interchapters, I will not focus primarily on students' final products. Instead, in the pages that follow I am most interested in students' attitudes and approaches toward the process of writing and how these change when they self-consciously embody their writing practices. Yoga teaches us that being on the path is what is important; the focus is always on the practice of a pose, a meditation or a breathing sequence, and not simply the outcome. Even so, there will be organic moments where students' reflections will lead me to their papers if only to underscore their changing ideas about writing. As will become clear, students' own reflective writings serve as a testimony that a focus on process doesn't preclude an interest in the texts our students produce.

While my opening depicts a healthy practice of *pranayama*, one easily accepted by my writing students and myself, this wasn't always so. When I started these breathing exercises with my students, I felt guilty. I worried that our breath work would compromise our time to complete the day's work. I was already devoting class time to teaching various yoga *asanas*, or postures, and adding another element seemed like it might encroach too much upon our learning routine. Even though I was committed to integrating the contemplative practices of yoga in my classroom, I didn't want my students to "lose" anything for the sake of their inclusion. So at first, I kept a close eye on my watch and tried to take attendance while I guided my students through their focused breathing.

This multitasking seemed to validate any time "lost." However, it problematically relied on a banking model of learning that implicitly valued multiplying skills over changing attitudes and also encouraged a rather hapless application of mindfulness—one that ignored the irony of attempting to cultivate awareness of the present moment by dividing my attention rather than focusing it. If I couldn't stop multitasking, what right did I have to ask students to? Was my move to take attendance while engaging them in *pranayama* any better than their attempts to watch TV or check Facebook while writing assignments for our class? Just as my students were slowly convinced of the effectiveness of mindful breathing through continued efforts, our classroom breathing gradually taught me the importance using contemplative practices in transformative as opposed to additive ways.

I was already witnessing a transformation of the learning culture of my classroom due to our practice. Breathing with my students was organically changing the pace of my teaching from a sometimes-frantic push to just-get-one-more-lesson-learned-reading-completed-writing-workshop-done to a more balanced and measured tempo. While I still felt the urge to push forward as the semester rolled along like a rock down a hill, I was learning the difference between acknowledging the presence of these urges and acting on them—much as I have learned to label my thoughts *as* thoughts in order to put them aside during my personal practice of sitting meditation. Indeed, the whole class seemed to adjust to our measured pace by more frequently entertaining silence as a strategy for thinking.

I often noticed my students, perhaps in part following my lead, pausing to reflect over ideas in comfortable, thoughtful silence. The silence that characterized our breathing exercises was spilling over into our other classroom practices, such as the discussions upon which I build my lessons. When I was quick to push students to talk before they were ready, they would often correct my lack of mindfulness with the simple query, "Can you give us a moment to think about this?" That this question was even directed to me by my students showed a *growing into* engaged silence and a newfound respect for it in our classroom; these queries were rarely, if ever, posed by students in my classes where such mindful breathing was not a part. *Pranayama*, it seemed, was teaching us all how important reflective, quiet thinking was in the writing classroom—and it was reminding me how infrequently such "active" silence is allowed to reign. Before bringing yoga and breathing to bear on the process of teaching writing, it didn't occur to me that students might need to be taught how to create generative and reflective silence within the space of our classroom, a kind of silence I value in my own writing process. This is a kind of silence students don't often entertain—largely because they don't have to since their teachers, peers or iPods easily fill in the void with voice. To construct a simple binary between the silence of mindfulness and the mindless voices of digital technology is not what I am after, but the increased volume and pace of our lives and, thus, classrooms is certainly ever the more reason to find means of refocusing on the present moment and reducing distractions, especially when we are engaged in the process of writing.

Since the beginning of that first semester of bringing *pranayama* into my classroom, I have come to see time for reflective silence and breathing during class time as equal in value to our time for discussion or in-class writing, and I participate as fully as I can while still prompting my students.[29] Mindful breathing and practiced silence, in other words, have become part of the work of my writing classroom, reminding me and my students how important it is for writers to cultivate a habit of reflection and a writing life characterized by awareness if we hope to use the writing process not only to communicate but also to learn about ourselves and the world in which we live. The attentive awareness that *pranayama* fosters applies equally to the goals of mindful living and also mindful writing, the kind of writing that can support an education vested in the principles of social justice and feminist pedagogy. It also helps create a strong contemplative foundation when paired with the "yoga for writers" practices I outlined in Interchapter Two.

EMOTIONAL FLEXIBILITY

Daniel Goleman is perhaps the best-known popular theorist of emotions in education and the workplace. Of great interest to educators are Goleman's theories of emotional intelligence, defined as "master[y of] the emotional realm" (1995, p. xiii). In his book, *Emotional Intelligence*, Goleman claims lineage from Howard Gardner's theories of multiple intelligences but faults Gardner for focusing on cognitive elements in his categories to the exclusion of feelings. Goleman describes emotional intelligence, calling it a subset of Gardner's personal intelligences, as an individual's awareness of her own and others' emotions toward the ends of self-control and the management of emotional encounters with others (1995, p. xiii). To prove the importance of emotional intelligence, Goleman spends much time working through case scenarios to highlight the benefits of addressing emotional abilities in the workplace and in education. He believes emotional intelligence acts a corollary to IQ so that while the latter is seemingly out of our control, working to "master the emotional realm" (1995, p. xiii) provides "a better chance to use whatever intellectual potential the genetic lottery may have given to [us]" (1995, p. xii). Within Goleman's economic model, focused on traditional understandings of success in work and school, emotions become a skill of the capitalist who seeks to profit as much from his financial relationships as his personal ones.

While widely popular, Goleman's term is too problematic for inclusion in contemplative writing pedagogy. First, although he admits that the emotional and the rational often work together in harmony, Goleman ultimately sees them as "two minds" that work as "semi-independent faculties" (1995, p. 9), which problematically gives the impression that comprehension can sometimes be devoid of emotion. This separation stands in stark contrast to a contemplative understanding of emotion as an organic form of our body's energy so that we can no more stop feeling than cease breathing (Iyengar, 2005, p. 82). Second, Goleman's theory tends to ignore difference and focuses more on promoting assimilation in a cookie-cutter, male-dominated world. His is a world of capitalists seeking to gain as much ground as possible, which unfortunately reduces emotional intelligence to the level of a commodity. Here, gender is ignored, often along with other factors of situatedness including class and race. Positioned within patriarchal capitalism, Goleman's term lacks attention to difference and diversity and is fixated on singular self-control of emotions, which are in turn feminized; he thereby constructs emotional intelligence as a site of masculinized social control where the gains lie in "creating 'smooth' and efficient worker relations" (Boler, 1999, p. 61).

In my last chapter, I introduced emotional flexibility as a means of approaching the work of feeling in contemplative pedagogy. Here, I suggest we trade talk of emotional intelligence for emotional flexibility. Goleman's term tends to denigrate emotional awareness to the level of a commodity, which can be deployed for capitalist gains. Because it refuses lineage from such troubled terms and springs instead from a tradition of yogic mindfulness that parallels feminist theories of connected and situated knowing, emotional flexibility is more hopeful and is self-conscious of embodied difference. Unlike emotional intelligence, which works within a genetic range bestowed upon us by fate or divine will (Goleman, 1999, p. xii), I approach emotional flexibility as a skill that can be cultivated, taught and learned—just as flexibility is taught and developed in the yoga studio. Indeed, by utilizing contemplative acts like *pranayama* as writing tools, my students grow to become writing yogis of their thoughts and emotions. That is, our classroom practice of mindful breathing helps my students develop emotional flexibility they can use to become more generative and reflective writers who are strong and resilient in the face of negative emotions and thoughtful and compassionate in their attempts to understand and utilize the meaning potential of feeling in their composing processes.

Our feelings, whether inspired by the ideas and memories about which we are writing, generated by the writing process itself, or produced by our body's responses and organic intelligence, energize our writing. I like how Iyengar, puts it: "The very word, inspiration, meaning both to breathe in and to grasp a feeling in the form of an idea, expresses the way the brain is charged during inhalation" and reminds us of the body's role in meaning creation (2005, p. 75). Iyengar accounts for what we might call felt knowledge after Sandra Perl's exploration of felt sense, or the "body's knowledge before it's articulated in words" (2004, p. 1). If Iyengar accounts for the ways invention is embodied, he does so by linking breath and emotion. According to yoga, focusing on the breath, *prana* or life force and energy, makes us attentive to our feelings (and thus able to reshape them). A focus on *prana* also stabilizes our mind by bringing it back into dialogue with our body, connecting us to the rest of the material world, in turn. In the simplest terms, *prana* situates us. And because *prana* is never still but rather flows between all material objects, this situatedness is dynamic. The very act of inhalation confuses boundaries between self and environment, insisting on an interrelatedness of all matter. Inhalation, therefore, literally opens us to new possibilities and ways of being and thinking that are in constant flux, teaching us patience in the face of change. Like catching our breath outside on a windy day or grappling with the evolution of meaning over the course of successive writing drafts, we must learn to be responsive to our ever-changing environments.

If situated knowledge, at its best, is attuned to the ways our social and material placement locates us in the world in particular ways, then *pranayama,* or the practice of focused breathing and awareness, represents how we both surrender ourselves to our environments and how we also exert ourselves on these environments as we filter them through our bodies, changing them and ourselves. By the deceptively simple act of breathing, then, my students learn to embody and enact the reflective and reflexive inquiry at the heart of the embodied imagination and to apply this to their own writing processes. As embodied imaginers, students join the social, emotional and bodily dimensions of knowing and of making meaning. Approaching feeling through the contemplative means that we understand it as, in part, sensational, a slowing heartbeat and steady hands, as well as emotive and conceptual, such as feelings of peacefulness and receptivity for the upcoming discussion and lesson.

Flexibility is the ability to bend without breaking; similarly, when applied to our emotions, it is the ability to balance the weight of our emotional responses and the need to accommodate others'. Yogis can only stretch as far as they can maintain balance; stretching without minding our own positioning will cause us to fall over. Mindful breathing helps us become aware of this need for balance and can teach us how to attain it through our bodies and exercise it in our mental and physical activities. To find this balance, or to become emotionally flexible, we must learn to pair the movements of extension and expansion. Iyengar explains that extension requires attending to our inner space and expansion requires reaching out toward others and the unknown (2005, pp. 33-34). The literal core of both acts is the center.

Respiration is a prime example of the coupling of extension and expansion, learned at the level of our bodies. During inhalation, our lungs expand and we bring the outside world into our body, allowing it to affect us, often in ways we may not initially predict. As we take in a breath, we literally and metaphorically take in and process the new, or that which we label as "other" because it exists outside of ourselves. If "[i]nhalation engulfs the whole body, expanding from center to periphery" (Iyengar, 2005, p. 75), then extension occurs in turn: "[d]uring exhalation, the tide recedes, drawing back toward the center" (Iyengar, 2005, pp. 75-76). For as we exhale, we move inward to our center, refocusing on the self, even as that self has been changed and shaped by the new breath circulating within our inner body until it too is released and the process begins again.

Mindful breathing, or *pranayama,* becomes a practice and a tool for teaching emotional flexibility in the writing classroom because it asks writers to pay attention to how the body feels and what the body does in order to develop writing habits that apply the strength and flexibility of the yogi to the writing process. Simply put, flexibility is achieved when writers can practice both self/inner- and other/outer- directedness and balance the two moves in their compositions and their composing processes. Here, the body is used as a hinge for new ways of *thinking* about writing and new ways of *doing* writing, or actually engaging in the process of composing. Instead of brains in vats, student writers in this paradigm are best understood as writing yogis, as body-heart-minds who use their physical beings as writing laboratories, or as lived sites for the practice and research of the writing and meaning-making process (enacting the expectation invoked in my epigraph). Mindful breathing thereby becomes an integral practice for instructors who want to forward embodied writing pedagogies that seek to rejoin the meaning-making potential of both thinking and feeling as they come together in the physical writing body. Imagining and enacting writing as a situated and embodied process by attending to the breath specifically invites students to think about how the body is integral to the composing process and how the relationship between thought and emotion shapes the tapestries of words and meanings writers create.

Emotional flexibility becomes a viable alternative to other pedagogical concepts of emotion as it authorizes feeling at the same time it considers those feelings in the context of outside perspectives, ambiguity and possibility. Indeed, traditional models of inquiry and critical analysis can be made stronger by being coupled with feminist acts of emotional flexibility. Too often the structure of "claim plus reasons" that rules academic argument seeks a kind of hollow closure and encourages our students to "play it safe" with surface-level topics that may or may not complicate, challenge or confirm embodied beliefs and values. Just as often there remains little room for students to explore ideas threatening to their identities, which are tied deeply to embodied beliefs and feelings. Within feminist contemplative pedagogies, however, emotion becomes not simply a subject of critical inquiry, but a process of inquiry itself. Teaching students to trace in their writing the entanglement of situated feeling and thinking and encouraging the development of emotional flexibility may prompt them to entertain new viewpoints seriously without the threat having to divorce from their flesh by capitulating to expert ideas or uncritically staying rooted in their own.

Even if it isn't standard practice to pay attention to the breath during the writing process, understanding meditative mindfulness as a primer for the learning process isn't as esoteric as it may have been even a few years ago. With the proliferation of yoga retreats for writers and the rise of contemplative education and organizations that promote mindful pedagogies in higher education such as the Center for the Contemplative Mind in Society, many educators have accepted the ways contemplation and mindfulness practice, such as meditation and *pranayama* (which is a kind of meditation focused on the breath rather than on a mantra), can be successfully deployed as part of a holistic learning process that links the body and the mind. Appreciating the breath "as it is" while learning to direct its energies toward where one wants it to be is pragmatic in the writing classroom, in particular, because it teaches students that they must start where they are, or that acknowledging their present reality is necessary to move forward toward new embodied imaginings which unify the body's desires and the mind's energies. On the page, these paired actions represent a fusion of the critical and the creative that characterizes the most socially-viable and personally-fulfilling kinds of writing our students can produce. Teaching mindfulness through the breath cultivates an environment of well-being that benefits teachers too. As Repetti notes, "[t]he professor who meditated with students is supporting not only her students but herself against teacher burnout and other ills that threaten motivation on a daily basis" (2010, p. 11).

WORKING TOWARD EMOTIONAL FLEXIBILITY

Encouraging students to approach their writing processes as embodied through the practice of *pranayama,* known to target the subtle body of emotions in yoga, helps them attend to their physical and emotional responses to writing. Mindfulness starts, after all, with the practice of paying close attention, a skill we deem necessary for successful writing. While we already insist writers apply such attentiveness to their subject matter, using the skills of close reading and analysis, we might also include increased awareness of the feeling body as the writing subject and the material origin of meaning. One way to respect the body as an epistemic origin is to become more aware of and responsive to our feelings as writers—"gut"/ ideational, psychological and physiological.[30] *Pranayama* asks writers to develop this corporeal orientation and trains them to attend to feeling via the breath.

Flexibility is literally the ability to bend without breaking; similarly, when applied to our emotions it is the ability to balance the weight of our emotional response and the need to accommodate others'. Yogis can only stretch as far as they can maintain balance; stretching without minding our own positioning will cause us to fall over. Likewise, I previously qualified emotional flexibility by insisting it included two complementary skills that encouraged equal application of reaching within and without in order to maintain harmony between balance and stretching. Here, I argue that the practice of mindful breathing engages student writers in and brings them through the paired skills of emotional flexibility, extension and expansion, which I developed in my last chapter. In *Light on Life*, Iyengar explains that extension requires attending to our inner space, or our center, and expansion requires reaching out from our center toward others and the unknown. The literal core of both acts is the center; extension moves inward to the center and expansion moves outward from the center (Iyengar, 2005, pp. 33-34).

These acts of emotional flexibility, needed to engage in an embodied rhetorical process, share much with what feminist Nira Yuval-Davis has recently called the "rooting" and "shifting" functions of transversal politics. Yuval-Davis credits feminists in Bologna, Italy for the cultivation of this democratic, feminist political practice based on three interlocking concepts: standpoint theory's reminder that because differing viewpoints produce varying bodies of knowledge, any one body of knowledge is essentially unfinished; that even those who are positioned similarly may not share the same values or identifications; and that notions of equality need not be replaced by respect for difference but can be used to encompass difference (Yuval-Davis, 1999, pp. 1-2). What I like about

Yuval-Davis' terms, "rooting" and "shifting" is their bent toward movement and their reflection of the skills of flexibility and awareness I approach from a yogic mindset. From Italian feminists Yuval-Davis introduces the concept of rooting as a reflexive knowledge of [one's] own positioning and identity" and shifting as "put[ing] [ourselves] in the situation of those with whom [we] are in dialogue and who are different" (Yuval-Davis, 1999, p. 3). Extension and expansion are the writing yogi's terms for rooting and shifting; flexibility is only achieved when we can practice both self/inner- and other/outer- directedness. That these acts are recursive and complementary insists on the importance of first understanding ourselves by locating our center so that an acceptance of where we are at any given moment is necessary to reach out toward the new.

This kind of centering isn't solipsistic since the very process of rooting in our center teaches us to shift toward an outside world of which we recognize we are a part, connected by our very materiality. This is because yoga sees all matter, *prakrti*, including that which makes up the body *and* the mind, as connected, exchanging dualities between body/ mind and self/other for a much more complicated understanding of intersubjectivity and connected beingness. From this viewpoint, acts of both extension and expansion are situated within a personal body but teach this body to be simultaneously inner-directed and outer-directed as it becomes aware of its connected nature by drawing within and reaching without. The emotional flexibility created by honing the skills of extension and expansion realize Haraway's behest that "[w]e need to learn in our bodies ... to name where we are and are not, in dimensions of mental and physical space we hardly know how to name" (1991c, p. 190) and may begin to name these spaces. These terms are also reflective of feminist themes of empowerment in ways a traditional vocabulary of emotions in education are not.

Mindfulness of and concentration on the breathing process can teach students valuable, practical lessons they can immediately apply to their writing. As we breathe, my students and I become more balanced in body and heart as well as in mind. Equanimity within the paradigm of mindfulness is best understood as a compassionate and balanced response, a meeting of extension and expansion, not an absence of feeling. Mindful breathing teaches students to embody this process of rooting in the center and shifting from the center, creating within them emotional flexibility they can apply to their writing. Receptivity and rootedness, like inhalation and exhalation, are parts of a whole process, necessary in equal measure for balance. Mindfulness of and concentration on the breathing process can teach students valuable, practical lessons they can immediately apply to their writing. In particular, students learn through our breathing exercises that effective writing sessions begin with responsiveness to their current feelings, which may position them as more self- or other-centered at any given moment. Only they can target which of our breaths will balance their emotional states, which is why the choice of breath documented at the start of this essay is so important. On an immediate and instrumental level, the choice of breath gives students a reason to become aware of their current energy level as well as how this relates to their receptiveness to the writing process. Students realize that they are faced with writing deadlines to begin drafting a new essay regardless of how energized they feel after a full day of classes and welcome ways of revving up their energy levels, no matter how atypical these methods may seem at first. As students begin to embody the lessons learned through mindful breathing to their thinking about writing, this developed equanimity translates into a more open engagement with outside sources and alternate viewpoints.

For instance, when the class I follow in my opening narration first attempted *pranayama* together, many students assumed that they were anxious simply *because* they were in class, so they used longer exhalations to calm themselves. They chose their breath based on what they anticipated feeling as opposed to listening to their bodies. As a result of using calming breaths when they were more tired than anxious, some of my students complained of sleepiness after our inaugural *pranayama* practice. As my student Johnny stated, "I found the breathing calming and relaxing, but almost too much to the point where I was lulled to sleep. I came out of the exercise feeling relaxed, but also with a strong urge to go to sleep." After a few more attempts, Johnny learned to "check in" with his feelings before choosing a breathing pattern. He noted in his blog that he stopped using long exhalations by default and began, instead, to analyze his feelings and scan his body. Johnny started working with the three-part inhalation to create energy and, therefore, engagement with his environment; after listening to his body, he found that was what he most needed. In navigating the consequences of his choice, Johnny learned two lessons: first, that he needs to pay attention to his body if he hopes to be an effective learner and writer, and second, that understanding and navigating his feelings is part of the work he must complete to this end. His breath became a means for these recognitions.

Johnny's experiences should also remind us that remaining open to new ideas is a task a peacefully attentive mind can handle with greater acuity than a foggy, sleepy one. Johnny's classmate, Ryan, reiterated this conclusion in his blog, stating that the three-part energetic breathing, "gives me ideas for writing, or simply refreshes me after hours of writing. After [breathing] breaks, I feel energized and usually have better ideas more readily than before breaks." Ryan links these "better ideas" to "the positive energy … the deep inhalations did give me …. Now I'm not going to lie to you, it wasn't a miracle cure. I didn't suddenly burst out full of energy, ready to conquer the world. But it did help." While not a "miracle" this "positive energy" was indeed a motivator. Ryan called up energy through his breath, channeling *prana* to give him the excitement, endurance and ideas he needed for writing.

In his comments, Ryan is likely referring to the effects of physiological coherence, which has been shown to result from contemplative practices like meditative breathing. "Correlates of physiological coherence include a regular heart rhythm, decreased sympathetic nervous system activation and increased parasympathetic activity and increased heart-brain synchronization (the brain's alpha rhythms become more synchronized to the heartbeat" (Schoner & Kelso, 1988; Tiller, McCraty & Atkinson, 1996; quoted in Hart, 2004, p. 31). In other words, the effects of the physiological coherence brought on by *pranayama* include the calming energy of focus as opposed to the jittery energy of caffeine since attentive breathing harmonizes the body and drops levels of anxiety. As Ryan's and Johnny's testimony highlights, students often begin to appreciate *pranayama* from an practical orientation rather than a philosophical one; the energy that mindful breathing gives them is a quality of our practice they value immediately—once hooked by practicality, deeper meanings have time to take root.

For instance, as Johnny's corporeal awareness grew as a result of practicing *pranayama*, he realized along with Ryan how breathing could not only help him monitor his states of feeling, but how it could also help him reshape those feelings. Johnny began to question the role of his entire body during our breathing exercises and after a few weeks, he relates increasing success in using *pranayama* as a writing ritual to how receptive he is to his full being and not only his breath while performing it:

> As we continued to practice the breathing exercises my goal has been to channel the exercises into becoming relaxed and energized at the same time. While I tried to adhere to all the instructions of the breathing, … I found myself still coming out the exercise more sleepy than I had entered …. With the last two practices I have felt myself become more and more relaxed and at the same time energized during the class exercise. I think I can attribute it to paying particular attention to my posture during the breaths …. Before I think I would allow myself to unintentionally slouch, or relax in the chair, contributing to my continued sleepiness from the morning. While focusing extra on my posture, I think I have been able to gain more from the exercise …. Writing after, I not only felt relaxed, I felt balanced.

My student's comment about posture is important for the ways it links the breath, body and mind together as they form his states of receptivity and rootedness. In slumped postures that allow the body to turn inward, Johnny found himself feeling so rooted he wanted to distance himself entirely from his environment through sleep. But when he concentrated on opening his body while focusing on breaths that continued this action, he felt energized and more connected to the community of our classroom and receptive to the learning process. These actions can explain why he feels a sense of emotional balance that he can take into the writing process after our practice.

As his teacher, I could see the effects of Johnny's growing mindfulness taking place in his blogs. Johnny's blogs at the beginning of the semester, those that correlate with a breathing practice that drew him further inward, were much more focused on pleasing himself as a writer. For instance, he states in these his intention of "getting out [his] true thoughts" as a writer and learning to have "no reservations about what I am writing." Later, as he attunes himself to his body and learns better emotional balance, Johnny's blogs contain more interest in audience and state his attempts to make his papers "easier to read for the reader" while still remaining interesting to him. While some of these growing concerns may be attributable to the workshops and peer reviews that were a part of our class, Johnny is also certainly embodying new attitudes about writing that grew as a result of composing with *pranayama*.

By the conclusion of our course, these lessons of balance and harmony permeated not only students' practical applications of the breathing exercises but also the ways they thought about the writing process. In a final class reflection, Mark noted that prior to our class he was reticent to open up to others. Mark isn't referring to shyness but rather a self-confessed inability to deeply listen to his classmates and to reflect on their differing viewpoints. He accounts for the new openness he felt at the conclusion of our course as an effect of his embodied awareness of the writing process developed through breathing exercises that engaged him in the acts of expansion toward others alongside extension toward his center.[31] Mark notes, "I can sense that in some ways I've grown more open .... Yoga and breathing meditation have helped my focus and made me more open. Hopefully both have made me a better, more intelligent person." The growth my student accounts for is holistic; in learning to balance his writing body and the outside world, he has grown flexible enough to respect his own ideas as well as to remain open to his audience and environment. The flexibility learned through yoga thus "becomes more than a physical attribute; it is transformed into a living metaphor" (Cohen, 2006-2007, p. 15). Mark senses that this growth is a gain for his "intelligence" which would give greater authority to his writing as well as his *ethos*, making him a "better" person and therefore, we can conclude, a more believable and persuasive writer.

What is interesting in Mark's reflection is his simultaneous attention to his developed "focus" on the self and the writing task at hand as well as his openness to others and foreign ideas. By noting both together, my student is actualizing the complementariness of extension and expansion. That he goes on to state in the same blogged reflection, "The learning that has occurred so far this semester because of our practice [of yoga and writing] has driven me to not take ideas and experiences at face value," testifies that he applied the lessons from our breathing practice to his writing. The strongest writing Mark produces, according to his blog, dialogues his "own ways" of being with "new ways of thinking."

Mark embodied this discovery with his final class paper, which he chose to write about deviance on campus. In his first draft, he argued that while underage drinking was an activity in which many college students participated, students who abstained would not be automatically socially ostracized for their decision. He spoke from his own experience of occasionally abstaining at parties when he had a big test the following day (he drank at other times). In talking with classmates about his ideas however, Mark encountered another student who passionately disagreed with him since she had indeed felt excluded because of her decision to abstain entirely from underage drinking. While Mark entered my class disdaining the practice of peer review because he felt his peers could in no way help him write a better draft, by the end of our class he sought out an interview with the student who disagreed and, without my prompting, used her as a source in his paper. He also asked me if the two of them could peer review with each other (I usually assigned pairs). Mark's final draft was a powerful mediation between his original arguments and his classmates' dissenting opinions. In it, he included his classmates' opinion that he didn't encounter ostracization when abstaining because he was already accepted as a "drinker" in his social circles: "I discovered that the barrier [between my experience and my classmate's] … was due to the bond alcohol creates between drinkers." Led by his breath, Mark didn't simply learn the power of using experience as evidence in his academic writing; he understood the necessity of analyzing his own experiences and putting them in dialogue with others' in order to build the most socially- and personally-responsible knowledge, knowledge that respects multiple "ways of being." As this example illuminates, these acts of emotional flexibility are metacognitive acts, acts of thinking about thinking, about writing and about being in the world.

Of course, for some students learning to take in less from the outside is crucial to their development of balance as writers. These students have overextended themselves in the past by being too receptive, causing them to lose their center as writers. These are the students that plead with us to read their ideas and tell them if they are "right" and ask us to just tell them "what we want" because they'll do whatever it takes to get an "A," if we could simply quantify that for them. In the past, I've found such students to be simultaneously some of my best writers and the hardest to teach because what I "want" is for them to take risks and to uncover their own views in their writing and not to regurgitate what they think mine are. Such unquestioning receptivity is a common problem for students used to echoing the thoughts of others and not investing the time to work through their own ideas either because they haven't prioritized their own thinking in fear of risking a "good" grade (preferring instead the "safe" essay) or because they are afraid their thoughts won't be merited against those of their teachers' or those espoused by other "experts." Writing that embodies the risky business of seriously considering another's ideas by taking them in and testing them against personal experiences and feelings is normally avoided. But, breathing exercises can help cultivate a mind more perceptive of the need for balance and can support a pedagogy that asks students to engage with their experiences. Mark's classmate, Megan explained that her balance directly resulted from what she learned from our breathing exercises and how she felt about her writing produced after these exercises: "Emotionally, I'm much more attached to what I write. I give very personal essays now in a way that I never did beforehand. I give essays that while reading back on [them], I don't feel alienated by [them]. I feel like they a part of me." Writing has become a means of developing self-awareness for this student.

Unlike Mark, Megan worried almost exclusively about her imagined audience. In early blogs, Megan wrote that it would be a sign of growth if she could begin to incorporate her own experiences and ideas in her writing and worry less about pleasing others and accommodating anticipated criticisms from her audience. After a semester of using *pranayama* to motivate and sustain her writing and increase her mindfulness, Megan did learn to become more responsive to her own concerns as a writer, according to her final, blogged reflection on her changed attitudes toward the writing process:

> This semester, my views on what it means to grow as a writer have drastically changed. Prior to [our class], writing was about pleasing an audience. Now, I have been searching more for what I care about and WANT to write about. I've also been focusing a lot more on my writing for exactly what it is. There's less comparison to the writing of those authors we read in class, and more comparison between my old writing style and new style. I think this is perhaps my greatest realization,

> because to grow as a writer means not to grow in the world as a writer, but to improve upon oneself and climb your own ladder ... I think that emotionally, I've got[ten] a lot more relaxed about writing through breathing, and that is growth.

Indeed, Megan's mid-semester writing marked a transition point for her as she found a link between the breaths she used to give her calm and confidence for her composing process and the voices she incorporated within her writing. For a mid-semester revision assignment, she wrote a triple-voiced narrative instead of a traditional, claim-driven argument because she felt it better represented her ideas, even if it risked shocking her audience—including me, her teacher. The essay that resulted was an extremely powerful one that narrated the extreme pressure female athletes face to stay thin and yet remain strong, a paradox my student explored with an academic researcher's voice and intermittently spoke back to with two additional voices: her own personal voice, which examined the changing thought process and confusions of a growing teenager, and the voice of popular culture as depicted by singer Rhianna's song, "Question Existing." The song both asks and genders the question of what it means to be judged for performance and image and champions living for oneself. The paper Megan produced thus embodied for her a lesson of claiming an authoritative voice so that I'd argue that while my student might not be able to write a multi-voiced narrative in her biology class, what she will have learned about rhetorical flexibility and the link between form and content will transfer to other classes, making her writing stronger there as well.

Every new language gives us new ways of thinking, and yoga does this for my students who are able to revisit and "re-see" the writing process as embodied by framing it within the terms of their bodies, emotions, movements and breaths. But what they gain isn't simply a new language, and what we gain as teachers isn't simply some Sanskrit to include in our professional writing; instead, these acts help us to talk with students in new ways about what it means to develop a writing practice, and how they might cultivate awareness of themselves as writers and meaning-makers and what the physical process of composing entails. That is, the embodied practice of *pranayama* urges students to plan generative, body-conscious methods of approaching writing and learning tasks, gives them a method of monitoring themselves as they move through their writing and provides a supportive system of stop-point evaluation more interested in intrinsic growth than extrinsic success, particularly in the form of grades. This shouldn't be surprising since *pranayama* is a means of metacognition itself, as it engages writers in learning to develop a conscious relationship to cognitive and emotional states that allows them to reflect on and to redirect their patterns of thought and feeling.

Breathing In Focus, Breathing Out Negative Emotions

Breathing not only teaches us balance by unifying the energies of self and the world but also helps us to concentrate on the present moment and to be attentive to our embodied needs in it. Meditation, whether on the breath, an intention or a mantra, has long been known to increase our powers of focus and concentration. As Iyengar states, "[w]atching the flow of the breath also teaches stability of consciousness, which leads to concentration …. The power of concentration allows you to invest your new energy judiciously" (2005 p. 72). By paying attention to our breath, my students learn to focus the energy of the physical and mental body, which can result in more productive writing sessions wherein they feel in greater control of the distractions that surround them. The stronger their powers of attention, the more likely it is that they will stay motivated to continue writing and the less likely they will be blocked by stress or anxiety.

While these are lessons individually felt, they are collaboratively learned. Because students do not always arrive on time to class and because we start with our breathing exercises, we've had to learn as a class how to deal productively with the interruptions not only caused by other loud classes heard through the thin walls of our room but also by our own members entering the room after we've started. When we first started our breathing exercises, my students would open their eyes to see who had entered; later in the semester the majority remained focused on their breath, a demonstrable effect of their learned attentiveness. Not responding to distraction is an act of agency and of choice that many students hadn't considered prior to the class. Our age of multitasking and my students' almost absolute reliance on technology hides the choice; the cell call may go unanswered and the blinking Facebook message ignored. Sam noted in her blog that before our class, she never thought about the importance of focus during writing, but that now she understands it and attributes her success to our practice of *pranayama*: "I would have never guessed that yoga … could help a person focus as much as it has for me. My new writing habits are definitely more productive that the ones in the past like watching TV and Facebooking." Part of what students are learning during these classroom moments is the difference between contemplative beholding what happens around us (noting the noise caused by a late classmate and then letting it go) and attaching to these events (peeking our eyes open to observe the entering classmate).

Students can apply these lessons to their own bodies as equally as to other bodies and their environments. Because breathing rejoins our body and mind and urges them to work together for a common purpose, it is a helpful practice for writers who find their own bodies sources of distraction when attempting to focus—a common problem. One of my students, Steven, said this:

> Through the last few weeks, I have been able to concentrate in English a lot more because of the breathing exercises. At first, I had a lot of trouble concentrating. My nose always itched, or I had to cough, or something like that. But after the first few times I learned to tune this out and concentrate on my breathing …. I am amazed at the changes that have taken place in my writing since I started this class. I now see writing as a lot more physical and I can really jump right into it with the right combination of breathing exercises and habits. I always look forward to using these methods while I write papers.

Deciding what distractions are enabling versus those that are disabling is a strategy students tell me they often use to stay focused on their writing when working in loud dorms or heavily-populated libraries on campus. Even in the library, where many of my students go to escape from the noise, is distracting for many. Some of my students were worried about peer judgment if they used *pranayama* in these public spaces: "I didn't like doing [breathing exercises] in the library at first, where I write most of my papers, because there are a lot of people there. I don't like closing my eyes, thinking about my inhalations, when others are around." The usefulness of the breathing exercises, however, tended to win out over the fear of peer judgment: "I don't mind [breathing exercises in the library] anymore, I just do it; I figure no one cares if I close my eyes for a minute. I mean there are people taking naps in the library, so really a breathing exercise isn't that weird or out of the ordinary there. I feel much more concentrated after the exercise so I'll do it in the library." The sheer number of students who reported performing *pranayama* in the library and other public spaces on campus testified to me just how much they valued the practice. *Pranayama* also encouraged students to re-evaluate the moments of the writing process when they weren't breathing. Another of my students, Cindy, noted in a blog entry that she took to listening to classical music on her iPod as a way of maintaining her mindful and peaceful state after completing breathing exercises. Cindy states that she "learned how important it is to develop and maintain focus this semester and to be aware when focus is lost. I didn't do this before." As a result, Cindy had come to my class with much frustration over writing. She was able to finally dispel this frustration through her breath.

Pranayama teaches writers that where the breath is, the heart will be as well. Cindy's response illuminates how the inability to focus can become both the cause and the source of the negative emotions of the writing process. If emotional stress pulls the body and mind in separate directions, then these moments of appreciating the breath teach students that to alleviate such stress, it is necessary to rejoin the body and mind; the breath becomes a vehicle for this. Iyengar tells us that "[t]he breath, working in the sheath of the physical body, serves as a bridge between body and mind" (2005, p. 73). Developing skills to channel the breath in hopes that the mind will follow can help writers cultivate successful strategies for navigating the demands of the writing process, demands that are often emotional and anxiety-producing for our students (and ourselves). Breathing mindfully can create positive feelings and cultivate a quieted and calmed consciousness, ready to create and problem-solve. We know this instinctively as we unconsciously take deep breaths before walking on stage, and we are even culturally reminded of the ways conscious breathing promotes focus when a friend encourages us to "just breathe" when we are in the midst of a trying situation, wondering what course of action to take.

Learning how to use the breath to refocus their emotional states is important for students who rush from one class to another, hardly giving thought to the ways their performance in one will impact their successful learning in other. For instance, leftover anxiety from a test taken in the class before mine can chip away at my students' concentration, leaving them to fret more over the correctness of their answers on that test than to learn a new reading or writing strategy during our time together. One of my students noted that these stressors, "like [his] math test … fall away when we breathe at the start of class," allowing him to apply a fresh mind and calmed emotional state to our classroom work. "After each exercise, it's like all my concerns for other classes evaporated for a while, and I could focus solely on English class. I feel not totally, but somewhat relaxed. It's a good start for the class and writing."

My student might be alluding to the ways *pranayama* helps develop mindsets that encourage awareness and acknowledgment of feeling in ways that are enabling rather than disabling. This is an applied skill of emotional flexibility. These "motivational mindsets" contain "scripts for dealing with competence-related setbacks" and "beliefs about the malleability of abilities as well as strategies and scripts for how to cope with inevitable setbacks associated with learning new and challenging things" (Roeser & Peck, 2009, p. 129). Feeling itself is not unwanted in the writing process, since with feeling comes motivation; what *is* disabling is when negative emotions like stress and anxiety overwhelm the writer. Because emotional flexibility centers on balancing inner and outer pulls, it can help writers "avoid reactive attachment [to feelings and thoughts] … allow[ing] us to observe the contents of our consciousness rather than simply being absorbed by them" (Hart, 2008, p. 33). In the end, this override of unthinking reactions to feelings doesn't so much invalidate their importance as it allows students to better understand them, and greater intimacy breeds emotional maturity.

> For example, instead of just seething with anger, the contemplative mind may allow a little more space between the anger [or other emotion] and us. We might both have our anger and also notice it—"Look at me being angry, what's that about?"—rather than simply being lost in the anger. (Hart, 2008, p. 33)

As students learn to first notice and them accept emotions, they become more metacognitively attuned to themselves, which can significantly impact their behavior and can encourage development of adaptive writing strategies that positively transform the process.

Intimate awareness of our feelings is therefore a key step in developing an emotional flexibility that will allow writers to develop coping strategies and motivational mindsets that help them overcome negative feelings. Highlighting how this process works by attending to the breath, Boris shared the following story on his blog:

> Today I was feeling really down on myself and felt as though I needed some type of pep talk. After going through the breathing routine on my own, I actually was able to re-energize myself. Afterwards, the work that I had done was so rewarding that I feel motivated to continue writing. Sometimes if I get myself in a slump I need to remember that just one exercise can help me feel better, help me to be able to focus on homework, and to make me want to continue. This is what's so good about the yoga I do, it has a day to day use ... [making me] emotional[ly] and mentally flexible.

Boris finds a source of resilience and "emotional and mental" flexibility through *pranayama*. Meditation and yoga has indeed been shown to "promote the construction of attributions to malleable source of difficulty and adaptive source of coping, particularly when confronting setbacks" (Roeser & Peck, 2009, p. 129). It is this adaptive coping Boris alludes to when he uses breathing as a soothing and calming exercise, much like a private pep talk. As in the discussion of anger above, my student is able to step back from his depressed mood which seemingly leaves him devaluing his abilities as a writer to ask, "What's up with that?" An alternative to seeking out assurance from another, an act that may be stilled by embarrassment, is a conscious channeling of positive energy using his breath.

This work to transform his mood increases his motivation such that my student feels emotionally-rewarded by the writing that follows.

These examples from our breathing practice show how yoga helps writers displace negative emotions and embrace self-compassion, which is a quality upon which the contemplative arts are built. In their article on the usefulness of contemplative pedagogy, Roeser and Peck argue that teaching students to exercise self-compassion helps them "take a kind, non-judgmental, and understanding attitude toward [themselves] in instances of pain or difficulty rather than being self-critical" (Roeser & Peck, 2009, p. 129). Given that so many of my students describe the writing process as painful and emotionally dissonant, such an attitude is essential in our composition classrooms. My students' testimonies embody the additional benefits of self-compassion for writers including greater feelings of confidence and competence and an increased, intrinsic desire for growth and improvement. Indeed, college students who exhibit self-compassion focus more on their learning and improvement as opposed to their performance in comparison to others. Studies have shown that students who have developed self-compassion are more likely to approach setbacks with a positive mindset and to correlate academic failures less with their sense of self-worth. Self-compassion is specifically correlated to students' understanding of moment-to-moment fluctuations in perception, taught by breathing exercises, and their increasing ability to become aware of habitual responses in order to redirect them and "create a calm and clear mental context from which to act" (Roeser & Peck, 2009, p. 130).

It is this calm and clear context my students describe: "I definitely used breathing exercises to help calm myself down. I get so stressed and generally I use crying as a release for the stress but in this case, it was breathing exercises that helped me to calm down and get my focus back when I got too overwhelmed. I think it worked … only one instance of tears!" And, "I used the breathing exercises to stay calm when things were not coming together as quickly as I planned. I knew that I was on the home stretch of finishing my portfolio so when I went to the library to finish up little things and compile it in the folder I thought it was only going to take me two hours, but it ended up taking me six." A longer than expected revision process, however, wasn't enough to derail my student: "I began to get frustrated knowing that I had other stuff I wanted to get done too, but instead of freaking out and getting frustrated like I did in the past I took deep breaths in and tried to stay calm." Breathing gives my students the ability to override their habitual and negative responses to feelings of stress and anxiety and helps them find control in their emotions, allowing them to redirect the energy of their feelings in more positive ways.

Attending to the energy of the breath attunes us to the flow of our emotional states because it requires us to be in the present moment and to judge ourselves less harshly as a result. In the end, increased compassion and mindfulness results in growth, according to my students:

> Using the breathing techniques, I think that emotionally, I got a lot more relaxed about writing, and that is growth. To be able to accept something as imperfect because it doesn't have to be perfect yet is growth. To be able to know that you can improve in the future, and to be able to find your own flaws and then smooth them over is growth … yoga helps to allow me to sit and concentrate and not need to constantly move. It allows me to sit. And write. And put my body into the paper. I can use all my senses to their fullest, and I can use myself and my ideas and my inclinations to truly write a good paper, one that shows my growth.

Acts of emotional flexibility are directly applicable to the writing process and can be learned through the practice of *pranayama*. Appreciating the breath "as it is" while learning to direct its energies toward where one wants it to be is pragmatic in the writing classroom, in particular, because it teaches students that they must start where they are, or that acknowledging their present reality is necessary to move forward toward new embodied imaginings which unify the body's desires and the mind's energies. Students who accept the duality of extension and expansion, learned first at the level of their bodies by means of their breath, more easily accept change and are therefore more likely to see writing *as* a process and complete multiple, global revisions; students who can better cope with ambiguity are more likely to respond productively to their classmates' opposing viewpoints, may be more open to multiple perspectives in other writings, more accepting of the situatedness of knowledge claims and less likely to ignore such complexities in their own writing; students who are able to face with coping strategies the negative emotions called up by writing will not only spend more time and energy on their writing but will also take more risks in their writing, leading to increased learning. On the page, the paired actions of extension and expansion represent a fusion of the critical and the creative, which characterizes the most socially-viable and personally-fulfilling kinds of writing our students—and we—can produce.

CONCLUSION: NAMASTE

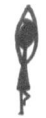

I breathe deeply; my students are about to finish their first "yoga for writers" practice with Holly and me, and they look happy and at ease. No one walked out, and I've enjoyed this more than I can put into words. I move with my students into a cross-legged position at Holly's request. We sit quietly for a moment, letting our practice sink in and acknowledging the ways it has subtly changed us in one short hour. Holly explains to my students that yoga practices end with bringing our hands in namaskar mudra, *which is a prayer-like position that aligns the hands under the breastbone. She instructs them and reminds me that we bring our hands together and say the phrase, "Namaste" as a way of honoring each other and ourselves. Holly asks us to say this Sanskrit word with conviction and with self-knowledge of what we can achieve when we are aware and acknowledge the union of our body, mind and heart. I recognize that it is this union that guides me, first as a yogi and now as a teacher.*

I bow my head forward and chant with the rest of my students, "Namaste."

NOTES

1. While some yoga poses will be explained and others visually represented within my text, many more will be only alluded to or omitted altogether for the sake of my narrative. I direct my reader to Appendix A for a copy of the handout I gave students after their first "yoga for writers" practice. While this handout does not include all the poses students learned in successive practices, it does represent the basic poses my yoga teacher and I used to create a foundation of yoga for students' combined yoga-writing practice.

2. Butler dismantles both sex and gender in *Bodies That Matter* as she attempts to address critiques of her earlier work, *Undoing Gender* (2004), in which she outlines her theory of gender performativity. A central premise of Butler's argument of gender performativity is that sex is not "a bodily given on which the construct of gender is artificially imposed, but ... a cultural norm which governs the materialization of bodies" (1993, pp. 2-3). In this book, I examine the limits of feminist theories of performativity and propose embodied alternatives by going to contemplative theory and practice. I am interested in writing pedagogies that utilize the strengths of both feminisms and the contemplative in my work.

3. I use this term throughout this book in a wide sense to include secular notions of the divine, which are often linked to the heart, the feeling center.

4. All student writing is taken from student-authored blogs in my first-year writing courses from 2009-2014. The students quoted in this book elected into my IRB-approved study. All students have been assigned pseudonyms.

5. This is akin to Belenky et al.'s connected knowing. Haraway defines the mutated modest witness' seeing as "passionate detachment," but I read it as connected, since her phrase is oxymoronic.

6. There are many reasons, then, why situated knowledge is crucial to Haraway's project. Like so many feminists of the third wave, she is driven to provide an alternative to whitewashed feminism, which takes women's experience to be homogenous without factoring in the differences of women everywhere, without accounting for crucial discursive and bodily constructions such as race and sexual orientation. The "woman" in the center of feminism has more typically represented the economically secure, heterosexual and generally normative white woman. Haraway's uneasiness over this homogenizing prompts her to be an early voice against claiming a singularity of women's experience, replacing it with multiplicity. Her preference for local, situated knowledges and tolerance for differential positioning will, in fact, establish a foundation for her latter theorizing of companion species based on kinship and relationality. As she proves time and again, closure is what should make us uncomfortable—a contemplative sentiment.

7. Haraway has indeed been taken to task over the differentiation of affinity and identity and has since taken pains to explain how it isn't so much that we can always choose our identities but that we can always choose to understand our inherent connection to others. She says in a recent interview: "I talked about kin as affinity and choice and people correctly pointed out that sounded too much like everyone rationally made choices all the time, and that's not good enough. There are all kinds of unconscious processes and solidarities at work that aren't about choice. Inhabiting "technobiopower" and inhabiting the material-semiotic configuration of the world in its companion species form, where cyborg is one of the figures but not the dominant one, that's what I am trying to do" (Haraway & Goodeve, 2000, p. 149).

8. George Lakoff and Mark Johnson build on previous work and approach the embodied mind through primary metaphors in language in their recent book, *Philosophy in the Flesh: The Embodied Mind and Its Challenge to Western Thought* (1999).

9. The differences between responses also highlight how important embodied notions of voice are as they determine who can speak against norms. The age and authority of the speaker, both of which are inexorably tied to the body, are differences that help to configure the right to speak.

10. This harmony could be compared to Mihaly Csikszentmihalyi's notion of the optimal "flow" experience. See his *Flow: The Psychology of Optimal Experience* (2008).

11. Sommers' essay is an echo of Tillie Olsen's "I Stand Here Ironing" as both seek to reflect on the nature of mother-child relationships. In Sommers' case, the "child" is her writing, certainly an embodied conception.

12. This is the problematic domain of the traditional modest witness (see my explanation in Chapter One). In the spirit of this critique, Hindman points out that positioning ourselves as modest witnesses in our writing confers the "right" kind of authority to our prose, legitimizing the ideas it espouses precisely because it divorces the writer from her material existence. Hindman explains how she is a victim of this epistemology, which is antithetical to the embodied writing she practices, in her article, [Mis]Recognizing Awesome Bodies.

13. Of course, the issue at hand is never as simple as calling expressivism "essentialist." There are many ways expressivism attempts to bridge or mediate the seemingly disparate positions of essentialism and constructivism. This mediation is a core thread running throughout Elbow's work, what he calls "embracing contraries." Here, I capitalize on how this embrace of contraries, because it allows for liberal-humanist notions of the self, is often collapsed into reductive essentialism. Whether or not this is a fair criticism of expressivism is not my focus here. I'm more interested in critiquing the idea that expressivist essentialism automatically reclaims the organic body.

14. Rosemary Hennessy in *Materialist Feminism and the Politics of Discourse* (1993) also argues that we need to see the interaction of the discursive and non-discursive.

15. I borrow and tweak Wendy Bishop's notion of a "teaching life" (*Teaching Lives: Essays and Stories*, 1997) for use in my classes. I've found that the notion of a writing life helps students classify the novel approaches to writing they encounter within contemplative pedagogy. And because it is rather open to interpretation from the start, this term allows students to define what a writing life means to them, giving students a stake in their learning processes.

16. The website, mindfuleducation.org, has a map of primary and secondary mindfulness education programs running in the U.S.

17. MBSR is a secular mindfulness practice and training program developed by Jon Kabat-Zinn. See umassmed.edu for information on MBSR and Kabat-Zinn's *Center for Mindfulness in Medicine, Healthcare and Society* at the University of Massachusetts. Also see Kabat-Zinn's *Full Catastrophe Living* for a detailed outline of this program. For an easy introduction to MBSR, I particularly recommend Bob Stahl and Elisha Goldstein's *A Mindfulness-Based Stress Reduction Workbook*. This book is an approachable guide to MBSR and fits well into larger discussions of learning and mindfulness in the writing classroom. It also provides a wealth of accessible practices for students and teachers that help address stress and increase mindfulness.

18. I am more interested in tracking students' habits and changing views of the writing process by examining their metacognitive reflections of writing than on the products they produce or their grades. As research on assessment shows, students' own perceptions of the writing process are equally-valid measures of their learning as exit exams or other product-based measures.

19. While Boler provides a holistic definition of emotion in line with my treatment of it here, she does prefer the term "emotion" to "feeling" while I use these interchangeably in order to underscore the social as well as bodily ways in which emotions are navigated and shaped. Boler chooses emotion as her primary term because it functions within our everyday, ordinary language and because she fears that the way feeling has been aligned with the sensational will restrict her attempt to bridge the cognitive, moral and aesthetic domains of emotion theory within philosophical psychology and philosophies of education (1999, pp. xix-xx). An example of the separation between feeling and emotion to which Boler alludes is Damasio's preference to denote the "private, mental experience of an emotion" as a feeling "while the term emotion should be used to designate the collection of responses, many of which are publicly observable" (1999, p. 42).

20. Haraway's term for interdependent species that shape each other in significant ways is "companion species." I discuss this co-constitutional model of subjectivity in my first chapter.

21. For my purposes, I will focus on Haraway's notions of human embodiment. For the ways in which our embodiment is complicated by animal-machine hybridity, see Haraway's Cyborg Manifesto.

22. Elsewhere, Bartholomae expands this argument regarding the dangers of ignoring the social construction of our ideas and feelings and claims, "it is wrong to teach late adolescents that writing is an expression of individual thoughts and feelings. It makes them suckers and, I think, it makes them powerless, at least to the degree that it makes them blind to tradition, power, and authority as they are present in language and culture" (1990, pp. 128-129). Bartholomae's classic critique highlights how emotion, conceived of as private, is put at odds with what is inherently social (language, power, authority) so that focus on feelings is necessarily a focus on the personal as foolishly removed from the public realm. But Bartholomae's critique must be bookended if we are to give weight to "emotion as a rhetorical, performative enactment" (Micciche, 2007, p. 42) which would ostensibly fit into his paradigm of social constructivist/ discourse community pedagogy. Even if emotions as experienced personally by an individual body, they are also social constructions, according to Micciche.

23. To be fair, Butler struggles with the materiality of the body and writes *Bodies that Matter* in response to the critical reception of her treatment of the body in *Gender Trouble*. In an effort to be responsive to her critics, she claims, "surely bodies live, and die; eat and sleep; feel pain, pleasure; endure illness and violence; and these 'facts,' ... cannot be dismissed as mere construction" (1993, p. xi). Even so, Butler does dismiss these facts of materiality when she later claims that "bodies only appear, only endure, only live within the productive constraints of certain highly gendered regulatory schemas" (1993, p. xi) and therefore lay no claim to materiality outside of discourse. To leave open the possibility of matter in excess of language is too dangerous for Butler who wants to question the organic nature of our gendered performances, a questioning that can be derailed with divisions between the naturalness of sex and constructedness of gender. Preferring closure on these debates, Butler ends up denying the materiality of sex along with gender, seeing them as cultural, linguistic performances. But, in my view, to lose the body to social construction seems no better than earlier paradigms wherein it was lost to naturalistic biology.

24. Micciche does acknowledge in her book that she is still developing pedagogical practices that invite the "rhetorics of emotion" into the classroom.

25. That feeling demonstrates the folding back or doubleness of our embodied selves has also been theorized by philosopher Merleau Ponty. Calling this the "double sensation" of feeling, he has said: "Between feeling (the dimension of subjectivity) and being felt (the dimension of objectivity) ... a gulf spanned by the indeterminate and reversible phenomenon of the being touched of the touching, the crossing over of what is touching to what is touched .... In the double sensation my right hand is capable of touching my left hand as if the latter were an object. But in this case, unlike an object, my left hand has the double sensation of being both the object and the subject of the touch" (quoted in Grosz, 1994, p. 100). The continuous flux of positions here, what Haraway might label our "differential positioning" within the

material world, shows the reversibility and thus companionate nature of the acts of feeling/ touching and being felt/ touched. This position of openness to the world does not mean that the subjects and objects of feeling are reducible to each other—the right hand is not the same as the left, but that they must always be understood as embracing one another (Grosz, 1994, p. 103). Ponty's notions of reversibility without reducibility correspond to Haraway's notions of companionate composers who too must be seen to make each other up in the flesh while retaining their own integrity. In other words, each is "significantly other" to each other.

26. This interchapter is an expanded and revised version of my article Writing Yogis: Breathing Our Way to Mindfulness and Balance in Embodied Writing Pedagogies, *Journal of the Assembly for Expanded Perspectives on Learning,* Vol. 18 Winter (2012-2013).

27. See Appendix B for a sample handout I provide students to guide our breathing exercises. While I introduce other *pranayama* methods to my students, this handout provides an overview of the core exercises we use together as a class.

28. The verbal prompts I've reproduced here are faithful to the same I used to guide my writing classes in meditative breathing. They represent an amalgamation of standard yoga exercises advocated in such books as *Yoga: A Gem for Women* (2002) and those taught by my yoga teachers, based on the traditions of Iyengar yoga.

29. At times, I ask students to try a completely silent breathing session without verbal cues from me. Because the majority of students express their preference for my guided prompts, I more frequently guide students. I understand their preference because I too enjoy guided *pranayama* in my own yoga classes. I am indebted, then, to many sources for the prompts I use to guide my students in contemplative practice.

30. Along with the tradition of yoga, I refuse the closure of neatly delineating between cultural affect, psychological emotions or physiological feelings. See Chapter Three for an in-depth theoretical discussion of emotion in contemplative pedagogy.

31. It may be worthwhile to note that while I talk with my students about centering and rooting in themselves as well as shifting outward toward others, I rarely use the terms extension and expansion in the classroom. While these terms are extremely helpful to me in my research because they allow me to work through the importance of these acts while drawing on the discourse of yoga, they become less helpful in demystifying writing or yoga for my students. I try to use as little of such jargon as possible with my students. For me, it is more important that they can engage in these acts and express them in simple, everyday language than it is that they can express themselves with the same rhetoric I use in my professional writing.

REFERENCES

Adler-Kassner, L. (2008). *The activist WPA: Changing stories about writing and writers.* Logan: Utah State University Press.

Ahmed, S. (2004). *Cultural politics of emotion.* New York: Routledge.

Anzaldua, G. (1999). *Borderlands/la frontera: The new mestiza* (3rd ed.). San Francisco: Aunt Lute Books.

Anzaldua, G. (2000). *Interviews/entrevistas.* (A. L. Keating, Ed.). New York: Routledge.

Baime, M. (2011, July). This is your brain on mindfulness. Shambhala Sun, 45–84.

Banks, W. P. (2003). Written through the body: Disruptions and "personal" writing. *College English, 66*(1), 21–40.

Bartholomae, D. (1990). A reply to Stephen North. *Pre/Text, 11,* 121–130.

Bartholomae, D. (1986). Inventing the university. *Journal of Basic Writing, 5*(1), 4–23.

Belenky, M. F., Clinchy, B. McV., Goldberger, N. R., & Tarule. (1973). *Women's ways of knowing: The development of the self, voice and mind.* New York: Basic Books, Inc.

Berlin, J. (1987). *Rhetoric and reality.* Carbondale, IL: Southern Illinois University Press.

Berlin, J. A. (2003). *Rhetorics, poetics and cultures: Reconfiguring college English studies.* West Lafayette, IN: Parlor Press.

Bishop, W. (1997). *Teaching lives: Essays and stories.* Logan, UT: Utah State University Press.

Bishop, S., Lau, M., Shapiro, S., Carlson, L., Anderson, N. D., Carmody, J., Segal, Z. V., Abbey, S., Speca, M., Velting, D., & Devins, G. (n.d.). Mindfulness: A proposed operational definition. Retrieved from http://www- psych.stanford.edu/ goldin/Buddhism/Mindfulness

Boler, M. (1999). *Feeling power: Emotions and education.* New York: Routledge.

Bordo, S. (1993). *Unbearable weight: Feminism, Western culture and the body.* Los Angles: University of California Press.

Brand, A. G. (1985–1986). Hot cognition: Emotions and writing behavior. *Journal of Advanced Composition, 6,* 5–15.

Brodkey, L. (1987). Writing ethnographic narratives. *Written Communication, 4,* 25–50.

Brodkey, L. (1994). Writing on the bias. *College English, 56*(5), 527–547.

Brown, K. W. & Ryan, R. M. (2003). The benefits of being present: Mindfulness and its role in psychological well-being. *Journal of Personality and Social*

Psychology, 84(4), 822–848.

Bush, M. (2011). Mindfulness in higher education. *Contemporary Buddhism, 12*(1), 83–197.

Butler, J. (1993). *Bodies that matter: On the discursive limits of "sex."* New York: Routledge.

Butler, J. (1999). *Gender trouble.* New York: Routledge.

Cavanaugh Simpson, J. (2009). Multitasking state of mind. In S. Maasik and J. Solomon (Eds.), *Signs of life in the USA: Readings on popular culture for writers* (pp. 469–471). Boston: Bedford/St. Martins.

The Center for Contemplative Mind in Society. (2002). Tree of Contemplative Practices. Retrieved from http://www.contemplativemind.org/practices/tree

The Center for Contemplative Mind in Society. (2013). Association for Contemplative Mind in Higher Education (ACMHE). Retrieved from http://www.contemplativemind.org/programs/acmhe

Cohen, J. B. (2006–2007). The missing body—yoga and higher education. *JAEPL, 12,* 4–24.

Cooper, M. (2011). Rhetorical agency emergent and enacted. *College Composition and Communication, 62*(3), 420–448.

Council of Writing Program Administrators, National Council of Teachers of English and National Writing Project. (2011). Framework for success in postsecondary writing. Retrieved from http://wpacouncil.org/files/framework-for-success-postsecondary-writing.pdf

Crick, N. (2003). Composition as experience: John Dewey on creative expressions and the origins of "mind." *College Composition and Communication, 55*(2), 254–275.

Csikszentmihalyi, M. (1990). *Flow: The psychology of optimal experience.* New York: Harper & Row.

Damasio, A. (1999). *The feeling of what happens: Body, emotion and the making of consciousness.* London: Heinemann.

Davis, J. (2004). *The journey from the center to the page: Yoga philosophies and practices as muse for authentic writing.* New York: Gotham Books.

DeLuca, G. (2005–2006). Headstands, Writing, and the Rhetoric of Radical Self-Acceptance. *Journal of the Assembly for Expanded Perspectives on Learning, 11,* 27–41.

DeMichelis, E. (2005). *A history of modern yoga: Patanjali and Western esotericism.* New York: Continuum.

Efklides, A. (2006). Metacognition and affect: What can metacognitive experiences tell us about the learning process? *Educational Research Review, 1,* 3–14.

Elbow, P. (1973). *Writing without teachers.* New York: Oxford University Press.

Elbow, P. (1990). Forward: About personal expressive academic writing. *Pre/Text*, 117–120.

Elbow, P., & Bartholomae, D. (1995). Writing with teachers: A conversation with Peter Elbow. *College Composition and Communication, 46*, 62–71.

Fleckenstein, K. S. (1997). Creating a center that holds: Spirituality through exploratory pedagogy. In R. P. Foehr & S. A. Schiller (Eds.), *The spiritual side of writing: Releasing the learner's whole potential* (pp. 25–33). Portsmouth: Boynton/Cook.

Fleckenstein, K. S. (2003). *Embodied literacies: Imageword and a poetics of teaching*. Urbana, IL: NCTE.

Fleckenstein, K. S. (1999). Writing bodies: Somatic mind in composition studies. *College English, 61*(3), 281–306.

Freedman, D P., & Holmes, M. S. (Eds.). *The teacher's body*. Albany, NY: SUNY Press.

Frey, O. (1993). Beyond literary Darwinism: Women's voices and critical discourse. In D. P. Freeman, O. Frey, & F. M. Zauhar (Eds.), *The Intimate critique: Autobiographical literary criticism* (pp. 41–65). Durham: Duke University Press.

Garland-Thompson, R. (2006). *Extraordinary bodies: Figuring physical disability in american culture and literature.* New York: Columbia University Press.

Garrison Institute. (2009). Envisioning the future of contemplative education: Garrison Institute symposium comprehensive report. Retrieved from http://www.garrisoninstitute.org/contemplation-and-education/ce-reports/728-envisioning-the-future-of-contemplative-education

Goldberg, N. (2005). *Writing down the bones: Freeing the writer within.* Boston: Shambala Publications.

Goleman, D. (1995). *Emotional intelligence: Why it can matter more than IQ.* New York: Bantam.

Grace, F. (2011). Learning as a path, not a goal: Contemplative pedagogy—its principles and practices. *Teaching Theology and Religion, 14*(2), 99–124.

Gradin, S. (1995). *Romancing rhetorics: Social expressivist perspectives on the teaching of writing.* Portsmouth, NH: Boyton/Cook Publishers.

Grossenbacher, P. G. & Parkin, S. S. (2006). Joining hearts and minds: A contemplative approach to holistic education in psychology. *Journal of College and Character, 7*(6), 1–13.

Grosz, E. (1994). *Volatile bodies: Toward a corporeal feminism.* Bloomington, IN: Indiana University Press.

Grumet, M. (2003). Afterword. In M. Grumet, *The teacher's body: Embodiment, authority and identity in the academy* (pp. 249–258). Albany, NY: SUNY Press.

Hanh, T. N. (1976). *Miracle of mindfulness: An introduction to the practice of meditation*. Boston: Beacon Press.

Haraway, D. J. (1991a). Cyborg manifesto: Science, technology, and socialist-feminism in the late twentieth century. In D. J. Haraway, *Simians, cyborgs, and women: The reinvention of nature* (pp. 149–181). New York: Routledge.

Haraway, D. J. (1991b). Reading Buchi Emecheta: Contests for "'women's experience" in women's studies. In D. J. Haraway, *Simians, cyborgs, and women: The reinvention of nature* (pp. 109–124). New York: Routledge.

Haraway, D. J. (1991c). Situated knowledges: The science question in feminism and the privilege of partial perspective. In D. J. Haraway, *Simians, cyborgs, and women: The reinvention of nature* (pp. 183–202). New York: Routledge.

Haraway, D.J. (1995). Toward a cyborg writing. In G. Olson & H. Giroux (Eds.), *Women writing culture* (pp. 45–80). Albany, NY: SUNY Press.

Haraway, D. J. (1997). *Modest_witness @Second_millennium. femaleman©_meets_oncomouse™*. New York: Routledge.

Haraway, D. J. (2003). *The companion species manifesto: Dogs, people, and significant otherness*. Chicago: Prickly Paradigm Press.

Haraway, D. J. (2004). *The Haraway reader*. New York: Routledge.

Haraway, D. J. (2008). *When species meet*. Minneapolis, MN: University of Minnesota Press.

Haraway, D. J., & Goodeve, T. (2000). *How like a leaf: An interview with Donna Haraway*. New York: Routledge.

Harkin, P. (1991). The postdisciplinary politics of lore. In P. Harkin & J. Schilb (Eds.), *Contending with words: Composition and rhetoric in a postmodern age* (pp. 124–138). New York: MLA.

Hart, T. (2004). Opening the contemplative mind in the classroom. *Journal of Transformative Education*, 2(1), 28–46.

Hart, T. (2008). Interiority and education: Exploring the neurophenomenology of contemplation and its potential role in learning. *Journal of Transformative Education*, 6(4), 235–250.

Hawhee, D. (2002). Bodily pedagogies: Rhetoric, athletics, and the sophists' three Rs. *College English*, 65(2), 142–162.

Higher Education Research Institute (HERI). (2005). *The spiritual life of college students: A national study of college students' search for meaning and purpose*. Los Angeles: UCLA Graduate School of Education & Information Studies.

Hindman, J. E. (2001). Making writing matter: Using "the personal" to recover[y] an essential[ist] tension in academic discourse. *College English*, 64(1), 88–108.

Hindman, J. E. (2002). Writing an important body of scholarship: A proposal for an embodied rhetoric of professional practice. *JAC, 22*, 93–118.

Hirschmann, N. J. (2004). Feminist standpoint as postmodern strategy. In S. G. Harding (Ed.), *The feministstandpoint theory reader: Intellectual and political controversies*. New York: Routledge.

Holzel, B. K., Lazar, S. W., Gard, T., Schuman-Olivier, Z., Vago, D. R., & Ott, U. (2011). How does mindfulness meditation work? Proposing mechanisms of action from a conceptual and neural perspective. *Perspectives on Psychological Science, 6*(6), 537–559.

hooks, b. (2000). *All about love: New visions*. New York: Harper Collins.

Howson, A. (2005). *Embodying gender*. Thousand Oaks, CA: SAGE Publications, Inc.

Iyengar, BKS (2002). *The tree of yoga: Yoga vrksa*. (D. Rivers-Moore, Ed.). Boston: Shambhala.

Iyengar, BKS (2005). *Light on life: The yoga journey to wholeness, inner peace and ultimate freedom*. New York: Rodale.

Kabat-Zinn, J. (1991). *Full catastrophe living: Using the wisdom of your body and mind to face stress, pain, and illness*. New York: Delta Trade Paperbacks.

Kalamaras, G. (1997). The center and circumference of silence: Yoga, poststructuralism, and the rhetoric of paradox. *International Journal of Hindu Studies, 1*(1), 3–18.

Karanikas, M. (1997). Spiritual empowerment in the technical writing class. In R. P. Foehr & S. A. Miller (Eds.), *The spiritual side of writing: Releasing the learner's whole potential* (pp. 157–166). Portsmouth: Boynton/Cook.

Kazan, T. (2005). Dancing bodies in the classroom: Moving toward an embodied pedagogy. *Pedagogy, 5*(3), 379–408.

Kirsch, G. E., & Royster, J. J. (2010). Feminist rhetorical practices: In search of excellence. *College Composition and Communication, 61*(4), 640–672.

Kroll, B. M. (2013). *The open hand: Arguing as an art of peace*. Logan, UT: Utah State University Press.

Lakoff, G., & Johnson, M. (1999). *Philosophy in the flesh: The embodied mind and its challenge to Western thought*. New York: Basic Books.

Lamott, A. (2005). Shitty first drafts. In P. Eschholz, A. Rosa & V. Clark (Eds.), *Language awareness: readings for college writers* (pp. 93–96). Boston: Bedford/St. Martins.

Langer, E. J. (1993). A mindful education. *Educational Psychologist, 28*(1), 43–50.

Langer, E. J. (1997). *The power of mindful learning*. Reading, MA: Addison-Wesley.

Lasater, J. (2000). *Living your yoga: Finding the spiritual in everyday life*. Berkeley, CA: Rodmell Press.

Lee, R., & Zolotow, N. (2002). *Yoga: The poetry of the body*. New York: St. Martin's Griffen.

Lv, F., & Chen, H. (2010). A study of metacognitive-strategies-based writing instruction for vocational college students. *English Language Teaching, 3*(3), 136–144.

Macy, D. (2008). Yoga Journal Releases 2008 'Yoga in America' Market Study. Retrieved from http://www.yogajournal.com/advertise/press_releases/10

Mairs, N. (1996). *Waist-high in the world: A life among the nondisabled*. Boston: Beacon Press.

Micciche, L. R. (2007). *Doing emotion: Rhetoric, writing, teaching*. New York: Boynton Cook.

Mindfulness in Education Network. (2014). Retrieved from http://www.mindfuled.org/

Moffett, J. (1982). Writing, inner speech, and meditation. *College English, 44*(3), 231–246.

Newkirk, T. (2004). The dogma of transformation. *College Composition and Communication, 56*(2), 251–271.

Olson, G. & Taylor, T. (Eds.). (1997). *Publishing in rhetoric and composition*. Albany, NY: SUNY Press.

O'Reilley, M. R. (1998). *Radical presence: Teaching as contemplative practice*. Portsmouth, NH: Boynton/Cook Publishers, Heinemann.

Paley, K. S. (2001). *I writing: The politics and practice of teaching first-person writing*. Carbondale, IL: Southern Illinois University Press.

Perl, S. (2004). *Felt sense: Writing with the body*. Portsmouth, NH: Boynton/Cook Publishers, Heinemann.

Repetti, R. (2010). The case for a contemplative philosophy of education. In K. Kroll (Ed.), *Contemplative teaching and learning: New directions for community colleges* (No. 151, pp. 5–15). San Francisco: Jossey-Bass.

Roeser, R. W., & Peck, S. C. (2009). An education in awareness: Self, motivation, and self-regulated learning in contemplative perspective. *Educational Psychologist, 44*(2), 119–136.

Robins, C. J., Keng, S-L., Ekblad, A. G., & Brantley. (2010). Effects of mindfulness-based stress reduction on emotional experience and expression: A randomized controlled trial. *Journal of Clinical Psychology, 68*(1), 117–131.

Royster, J. J. (2000). *Traces of a stream: Literacy and social change among African American women*. Pittsburg, PA: University of Pittsburg Press.

Rudrauf, D, Lutz, A., Cosmelli, D., Lachaux, J-P., & Le Van Quyen, M. (2003).

From autopoiesis to neurophenomenology: Francisco Varela's exploration of the biophysics of being. *Bio Res, 36*, 21–59.

Sanchez, R. (2012). Outside the text: Retheorizing empiricism and identity. *College English, 74*(3), 234–246.

Shusterman, R. (2008). *Body consciousness: A philosophy of mindfulness and somaesthetics*. New York: Cambridge University Press.

Siegel, D. J. (2007). *The mindful brain: Reflection and attunement in the cultivation of well-being*. New York: W. W. Norton & Company.

Simmer-Brown, J., & Grace, F. (Eds.). (2011). *Meditation and the classroom: Contemplative pedagogy for religious studies*. Albany, New York: SUNY Press.

Skorczewski, D. (2000). "Everybody has their own ideas": Responding to cliché in student writing. *College Composition and Communication, 52*(2), 220–239.

Smalley, S. L., & Winston, D. (2010). *Fully present: The science, art and practice of mindfulness*. Philadelphia, PA: Da Capo Press.

Spigelman, C. (2004). *Personally speaking: Experience as evidence in academic discourse*. Carbondale, IL: Southern Illinois University Press.

Stahl, B., & Goldstein, E. (2010). *A mindfulness-based stress reduction workbook*. Oakland, CA: New Harbinger Publications.

Tannen, D. (1998). *The argument culture: moving from debate to dialogue*. New York: Random House.

Teachers College Record. Contemplative practices and education. Special Issue. New York: Teachers College, Columbia University.

Tirch, D. D. (2010). Mindfulness as a context for the cultivation of compassion. *International Journal of Cognitive Therapy, 3*(2), 113–123.

Tompkins, J. (1996). *A life in school: What the teacher learned*. New York: Addison-Wesley Publishing Company, Inc.

Tompkins, J. (1987). Me and my shadow. *New Literary History, 19*(1), 169–178.

Worsham, L. (2001). Going postal: Pedagogic violence and the schooling of emotion. In H. A. Giroux & K. Myrsiades (Eds.), *Beyond the corporate university: Culture and pedagogy in the new millennium* (pp. 229–265). Landham, MD: Rowman & Littlefield Publishers.

Winans, A. E. (2012). Cultivating critical emotional literacy: Cognitive and contemplative approaches to engaging difference. *College English, 75*(2), 150–170.

Yoga sutras of patanjali. (2009). (E. Bryant, Trans.). New York: North Point Press.

Yuval-Davis, N., & Stoetzler, M. (2002). Standpoint theory, situated knowledge and the situated imagination. *Feminist Theory, 3*(3), 315–333.

Yuval-Davis, N. (1999). What is "transversal politics"? *Soundings, 12*, 94–98.

Zajonc, A. (2010). Contemplative pedagogy: A quiet revolution in higher education. In K. Kroll (Ed.), *Contemplative teaching and learning: New directions for community colleges* (No. 151, pp. 83–94). San Francisco: Jossey-Bass.

APPENDIX A: YOGA ASANA HANDOUT

Iyengar Yoga for Writers[*]

Before writing/at the beginning of yoga/ writing practice
- Set an intention for your practice
- Bring attention to the breath

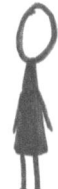

Mountain Pose

When you get stuck, can't concentrate or need a break
- Upward Salute: from standing, extend your arms overhead
- Upward Bound Fingers: from standing, interlace your fingers, turn your palms away from you and stretch your arms overhead

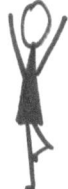   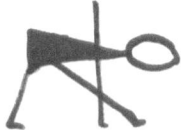

Tree Pose   Triangle Pose

---

* This handout was co-composed by the author and her certified Iyengar yoga instructor, Holly, who graciously helped teach the "yoga for writers" practices referenced in this interchapter. This handout does not represent all the variations of yoga taught to writing students, but does show one format introduced at the start of the semester.

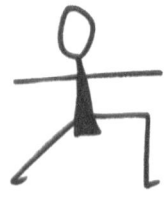 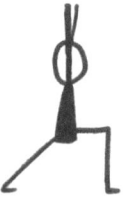

Warrior 2 Warrior 1

<u>Benefits</u>
Physical: Create stability, develop strength and stamina
Mental/Emotional: Improve concentration and focus

When you need to think through counter-arguments or expand your perspective

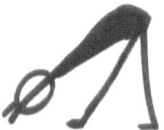 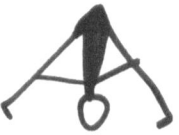

Pyramid Pose   Wide Leg Standing Forward Bend

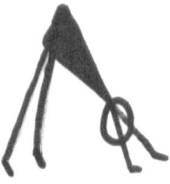 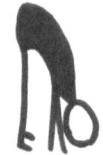

Downward-Facing Dog   Standing Forward Bend

<u>Benefits</u>
Physical: As above and relieve fatigue
Mental/Emotional: Build mental stability and clarity

Appendix A

When you come back to revise a piece of writing

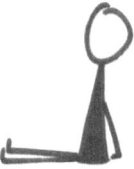

Staff Pose

- Variation: Extend arms up overhead, then bend forward from the hip crease and hold the outer edges of the feet.

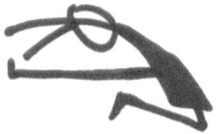

Head-to-Knee Forward Bend

- Sitting upright, extend arms overhead, then fold forward from the hip crease and hold the outer edges of the foot, then bend the elbows up and out to the sides to take the abdomen and the chest to the thigh and the forehead and chin to the shin.

Benefits
Physical: Lengthen the hamstrings; create extension in the spinal column, open the body; relive fatigue; relieve stress
Mental/Emotional: Relieve fatigue; quiet the mind

Ending a writing session

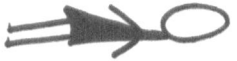

Final Relaxation Pose

- Lie down on the floor and rest deeply.
- Breathing I, II, III (I=becoming aware of the breath, even breathing; II=deepening the exhalation, normal inhalation III= deepening the inhalation, normal exhalation)

Benefits
Physical/Mental/Emotional: Encourage integration and acceptance.

APPENDIX B:
YOGA PRANAYAMA HANDOUT

WRITER'S YOGA BREATHING*

Sit up straight in your chair, feet planted firmly on the ground. No cross legs or slouching. Neck in line with back in line with tailbone. You should be alert but also comfortable.

Proceed slowly and with purpose through the next steps

Close your eyes softly. Bring the lids together, touching but not squeezing them, so you feel the horizon of your sealed eyelids. Let the pupils of your eyes begin to migrate slowly toward the back of your head.

Scan your body for tension and release it.

Tune your ears inward, and begin to listen to the sound of your own breath.
- Follow your exhalations to their natural end, without closing in the walls of your throat. Keep your abdomen relaxed, shoulders melting away from your ears on the inhalations, chest lifting away from your thighs on the exhalations. **(Continue this slow, soft, quiet breathing).**

Pay attention to your breath, the inhalations and exhalations, without trying to change them. Let your breath be perfect, just as it is in this moment. If your thoughts pull you away from your breath, gently guide them back to your breath. **(Stay here for a few moments).**

---

* This handout is inspired by Holly, my yoga teacher discussed within these pages, and the practices and phrases she used in my classes with her. As we tend to do, I've used my experiences in her classes as a yoga student as inspiration for my own teaching methods and prompts here. Holly's own techniques can often be traced back to the practices outlined in *Yoga: A Gem for Women* (2002).

Now, based on how you are feeling today, choose which breath is right for you:
- If you are tired, work on our three-part inhalation, sharply inhaling to your lower, middle, then upper ribs. Pause after each inhale and once you reach the top ribs, release your breath in a steady exhale.
- If you are stressed and anxious, begin to deepen your exhalations, so they become longer than your inhalations. See your inhalations as "small" and your exhalations as "big." You can try inhaling for three slow counts and exhaling for five slow counts, if this helps.
- If you are feeling fairly balanced already, simply concentrate on smoothing out your inhalations and exhalations, making them soft and quiet."

Allow your inhalations to give you energy and your exhalations to expel all the worries and stresses of your day. Find peace in your breath. **(Stay here for a few moments).**

Keeping your eyes closed, let your breathing return to normal, but keep it smooth and calm. Pay attention to your feelings of calm and steadiness. Resolve to carry these into the rest of your day. **(Stay here for a few moments).**

Now, take a minute to set an intention for yourself. Your intention could be grounded in the learning goals you have for our class or for all of your classes today. It may even encompass your social and academic lives. What do you hope to accomplish today or this week in your writing, your living, your learning?

Slowly open your eyes.

Opening your notebook, take a minute to record your feelings after this breathing exercise.

ABOUT THE AUTHOR

Christy I. Wenger is an Assistant Professor of English, Rhetoric and Composition at Shepherd University in Shepherdstown, West Virginia. At Shepherd, Wenger directs the Writing and Rhetoric program and was recently awarded the Annette H. Murphy Excellence Award, which recognizes meritorious teaching. Her research has focused on the intersections between feminisms, contemplative traditions and composition. In addition to bringing her own practice of yoga into the classroom, she has partnered with local yoga instructors to create learning communities between first-year experience courses and first-year writing courses and her research has benefited greatly from the generosity of her yoga community. Her work on the materiality of teaching and the value of contemplative pedagogy and administration has previously appeared in journals such as *WPA: Writing Program Administration, English Teaching: Practice and Critique,* and *JAEPL,* and has been shared at conferences held by the College Composition and Communication, the Rhetorical Society of America and the Association for the Contemplative Mind in Higher Education, among others. She serves as blog editor and board member for the Assembly for the Expanded Perspectives on Learning, an organization of NCTE that allows her to connect with other compositionists interested in alternative pedagogies. Her additional scholarly interests include feminist writing program administration, digital pedagogy and feminist disability studies.

www.ingramcontent.com/pod-product-compliance
Lightning Source LLC
Chambersburg PA
CBHW021857230426
43671CB00006B/418